Meniere's Disease

Guest Editors

JEFFREY P. HARRIS, MD, PhD
QUYEN T. NGUYEN, MD, PhD

OTOLARYNGOLOGIC CLINICS OF NORTH AMERICA

www.oto.theclinics.com

October 2010 • Volume 43 • Number 5

SAUNDERS an imprint of ELSEVIER, Inc.

W.B. SAUNDERS COMPANY

A Division of Elsevier Inc.

1600 John F. Kennedy Boulevard • Suite 1800 • Philadelphia, Pennsylvania 19103-2899

http://www.theclinics.com

OTOLARYNGOLOGIC CLINICS OF NORTH AMERICA Volume 43, Number 5
October 2010 ISSN 0030-6665, ISBN-13: 978-1-4377-2476-9

Editor: Joanne Husovski
Developmental Editor: Jessica Demetriou

Otolaryngologic Clinics of North America (ISSN 0030-6665) is published bimonthly by Elsevier, Inc., 360 Park Avenue South, New York, NY 10010-1710. Months of issue are February, April, June, August, October, and December. Business and Editorial Offices: 1600 John F. Kennedy Blvd., Suite 1800, Philadelphia, PA 19103-2899. Customer Service Office: 6277 Sea Harbor Drive, Orlando, FL 32887-4800. Periodicals postage paid at New York, NY and additional mailing offices. Subscription prices is $290.00 per year (US individuals), $527.00 per year (US institutions), $142.00 per year (US student/resident), $382.00 per year (Canadian individuals), $662.00 per year (Canadian institutions), $429.00 per year (international individuals), $662.00 per year (international institutions), $219.00 per year (international & Canadian student/resident). Foreign air speed delivery is included in all *Clinics'* subscription prices. All prices are subject to change without notice. **POSTMASTER:** Send address changes to *Otolaryngologic Clinics of North America*, Elsevier Health Sciences Division, Subscription Customer Service, 3251 Riverport Lane, Maryland Heights, MO 63043. **Telephone: 1-800-654-2452 (U.S. and Canada); 314-447-8871 (outside U.S. and Canada). Fax: 314-447-8029. E-mail: journalscustomerservice-usa@elsevier.com (for print support); journalsonlinesupport-usa@elsevier.com (for online support).**

Reprints. For copies of 100 or more of articles in this publication, please contact the Commercial Reprints Department, Elsevier Inc., 360 Park Avenue South, New York, NY 10010-1710. Tel.: 212-633-3812; Fax: 212-462-1935; E-mail: reprints@elsevier.com.

Otolaryngologic Clinics of North America is also published in Spanish by McGraw-Hill Interamericana Editores S.A., P.O. Box 5-237, 06500 Mexico D.F., Mexico.

Otolaryngologic Clinics of North America is covered in *MEDLINE/PubMed (Index Medicus), Current Contents/Clinical Medicine, Excerpta Medica, BIOSIS, Science Citation Index,* and *ISI/BIOMED.*

Printed and bound by CPI Group (UK) Ltd, Croydon, CR0 4YY

Transferred to Digital Print 2011

Contributors

GUEST EDITORS

JEFFREY P. HARRIS, MD, PhD, FACS
Chief of Otolaryngology/Head and Neck Surgery, Professor of Surgery/Otology and
Neurological Surgery, University of California San Diego School of Medicine;
Editor-in-Chief, Audiology & Neurotology; Staff Surgeon, VA San Diego Medical Center,
San Diego, California

QUYEN T. NGUYEN, MD, PhD
Director, Facial Nerve Clinic; Assistant Professor of Surgery, Otology/Neurotology
Section, Division of Head and Neck Surgery, Department of Surgery, University
of California San Diego, San Diego, California

AUTHORS

MEREDITH E. ADAMS, MD
Assistant Professor, Otology and Neurotology, Department of Otolaryngology–Head
and Neck Surgery, University of Minnesota, Minneapolis, Minnesota

YURI AGRAWAL, MD
Department of Otolaryngology–Head and Neck Surgery, The Johns Hopkins University
School of Medicine, Baltimore, Maryland

THOMAS H. ALEXANDER, MD, MHS
Neurotology Fellow, Division of Otolaryngology–Head and Neck Surgery, University
of California San Diego, San Diego, California

JAMES C. ANDREWS, MD
Department of Surgery, Northridge Hospital Medical Center, Northridge, California;
Department of Surgery, Sepulveda Veterans Administration Hospital, Sepulveda,
California; Clinical Professor of Surgery, David Geffen School of Medicine at UCLA,
Los Angeles, California

KAREN I. BERLINER, PhD
Clinical Studies Department, House Ear Institute, Los Angeles, California

MARCO CAVERSACCIO, MD
Professor, Department of Otorhinolaryngology, Head and Neck Surgery, Inselspital,
University of Berne, Berne, Switzerland

M. JENNIFER DEREBERY, MD, FACS
House Clinic and Clinical Studies, Department of House Ear Institute; Clinical Professor
of Otolaryngology, USC Keck School of Medicine, Los Angeles, California

JONI DOHERTY, MD, PhD
Division of Otolaryngology–Head and Neck Surgery, University of California San Diego,
San Diego, California

WILLIAM P.R. GIBSON, MD, FRCS, FRACS
Professor of Otolaryngology, The University of Sydney, New South Wales, Australia

SIMON L. GREENBERG, MB BS (Hons), FRACS
Neurotology and Skull Base Fellow, Department of Otolaryngology–Head and Neck Surgery, Sunnybrook Health Sciences Centre, University of Toronto, Toronto, Ontario, Canada

KIM R. GOTTSHALL, PhD
Department of Otolaryngology, Naval Medical Center San Diego, Spatial Orientation Center, San Diego, California

JEFFREY P. HARRIS, MD, PhD, FACS
Chief of Otolaryngology/Head and Neck Surgery, Professor of Surgery/Otology and Neurological Surgery, University of California San Diego School of Medicine; Editor-in-Chief, Audiology & Neurotology; Staff Surgeon, VA San Diego Medical Center, San Diego, California

RUDOLF HÄUSLER, MD
Professor, Department of Otorhinolaryngology, Head and Neck Surgery, Inselspital, University of Berne, Berne, Switzerland

KATHERINE D. HEIDENREICH, MD
Assistant Professor, Division of Otology and Neurotology, Department of Otolaryngology–Head and Neck Surgery, University of Michigan Health System, Ann Arbor, Michigan

CAPT. MICHAEL E. HOFFER, MD, MC, USN
Department of Otolaryngology, Naval Medical Center San Diego, Spatial Orientation Center, San Diego, California

VICENTE HONRUBIA, MD, DSc
Department of Surgery, Northridge Hospital Medical Center, Northridge, California; Emeritus Professor of Surgery, David Geffen School of Medicine at UCLA, Los Angeles, California

PAUL R. KILENY, PhD
Professor and Director, Division of Audiology and Electrophysiology, Department of Otolaryngology–Head and Neck Surgery, University of Michigan Health System, Ann Arbor, Michigan

LLOYD B. MINOR, MD
Department of Otolaryngology–Head and Neck Surgery, The Johns Hopkins University School of Medicine, Baltimore, Maryland

SHINJI NAGANAWA, MD
Professor, Department of Radiology, Nagoya University School of Medicine, Nagoya, Japan

TSUTOMU NAKASHIMA, MD
Professor, Department of Otolaryngology, Nagoya University School of Medicine, Nagoya, Japan

JULIAN M. NEDZELSKI, MD, FRCSC
Professor Emeritus, Department of Otolaryngology–Head and Neck Surgery, Sunnybrook Health Sciences Centre, University of Toronto, Toronto, Ontario, Canada

STEFAN K. PLONTKE, MD
Department of Otorhinolaryngology, Head and Neck Surgery, Tübingen Hearing Research Center (THRC), University of Tubingen, Germany

DENNIS POE, MD
Associate Professor, Department of Otolaryngology, University of Tampere, Tampere, Finland; Department of Otology and Laryngology, Harvard Medical School, Boston, Massachusetts

ILMARI PYYKKÖ, MD
Professor, Department of Otolaryngology, University of Tampere, Tampere, Finland

STEVEN D. RAUCH, MD
Professor, Otology and Laryngology, Harvard Medical School, Massachusetts Eye and Ear Infirmary, Boston, Massachusetts

ALEC N. SALT, PhD
Department of Otolaryngology, Washington University School of Medicine, St Louis, Missouri

KAREN B. TEUFERT, MD
House Ear Institute, Los Angeles, California

LT. SHELBY G. TOPP, MD, MC, USN
Department of Otolaryngology, Naval Medical Center San Diego, San Diego, California

DOMINIQUE VIBERT, MD
Professor, Department of Otorhinolaryngology, Head and Neck Surgery, Inselspital, University of Berne, Berne, Switzerland

JEFFREY T. VRABEC, MD
Associate Professor, Bobby R. Alford Department of Otolaryngology–Head and Neck Surgery Baylor College of Medicine, Houston, Texas

JING ZOU, MD
Associate Professor, Department of Otolaryngology, University of Tampere, Tampere, Finland

ADVISORS TO OTOLARYNGOLOGIC CLINICS 2010

SAMUEL BECKER, MD
Becker Nose and Sinus Center; Voorhees, New Jersey

DAVID HAYNES, MD
Vanderbilt University; Nashville, Tennessee

BRIAN KAPLAN, MD
Ear, Nose, and Throat Associates; Baltimore, Maryland

JOHN KROUSE, MD, PhD
Temple University Medicine; Philadelphia, Pennsylvania

ANIL KUMAR LALWANI, MD
New York University Langone Medical Center; New York, New York

ARLEN MEYERS, MD, MBA
University of Colorado; Denver, Colorado

MATTHEW RYAN, MD
University of Texas Southwestern Medical Center, Dallas, Texas

RALPH TUFANO, MD
Johns Hopkins Medicine; Baltimore, Maryland

Contents

The burden of Meniere's syndrome (MS) is substantial, especially when considering the significant impact on the quality of life of those affected. Reported estimates of incidence and prevalence have varied widely due to methodological differences between studies, changes in criteria for diagnosis of MS, and differences in populations studied. Reported prevalence rates for MS range from 3.5 per 100,000 to 513 per 100,000. A recent study using health claims data for more than 60 million patients in the United States found prevalence of 190 per 100,000 with a female:male ratio of 1.89:1. The prevalence of MS increases with increasing age.

It is well established that endolymphatic hydrops plays a role in Meniere's disease, even though the precise role is not fully understood and the presence of hydrops in the ear does not always result in symptoms of the disease. It nevertheless follows that a scientific understanding of how hydrops arises, how it affects the function of the ear, and how it can be manipulated or reversed could contribute to the development of effective treatments for the disease. Measurements in animal models in which endolymphatic hydrops has been induced have given numerous insights into the relationships between hydrops and other pathologic and electrophysiological changes, and how these changes influence the function of the ear. The prominent role of the endolymphatic sac in endolymph volume regulation, and the cascade of histopathological and electrophysiological changes that are associated with chronic endolymphatic hydrops, have now been established. An increasing number of models are now available that allow specific aspects of the interrelationships to be studied. The yclical nature of Meniere's symptoms gives hope that treatments can be developed to maintain the ear in permanent state of remission, possibly by controlling endolymphatic hydrops, thereby avoiding the rogressive damage and secondary pathologic changes that may also contribute to the patient's symptoms.

Meniere's syndrome is an inner ear disorder characterized by spontaneous attacks of vertigo, fluctuating low-frequency sensorineural hearing loss, aural fullness and tinnitus. When the syndrome is idiopathic and cannot be attributed to any other cause (eg, syphilis, immune-mediated inner ear disease, surgical trauma), it is referred to as Meniere's disease. This article reviews the physiologic effects of Meniere's disease on vestibular function, as measured by caloric, head impulse, and vestibular-evoked myogenic potential testing.

In this article, the present state of the art with respect to audiovestibular testing for Meniere's disease (MD) is reviewed. There is no gold standard for MD diagnosis, and the classic dictum is that even the "best" tests yield positive results in only two-thirds of patients with MD. Still, we advocate the use and further investigation of advanced audiovestibular testing in patients with MD in an attempt to answer the questions that confront any clinician who cares for patients with audiovestibular symptoms.

Meniere's disease is one of the most fascinating and most vexing of all clinical conditions encountered by the otolaryngologist. Operationally speaking, a Meniere's ear is a fragile ear. In fact, Meniere's disease can and should be redefined as a degenerating inner ear that has impairment of one or more homeostatic systems, resulting in instability of hearing and balance function. This updated definition is a valuable guide to the clinical epidemiology and presentation of Meniere's disease and to understanding the effects of conservative treatments. In the absence of a definitive test for Meniere's disease, the greatest challenge for the clinician may be differentiating this condition from migraine. Ultimately, Meniere's vertigo attacks are controllable in more than 99% of cases, but hearing loss and other auditory symptoms tend to be unresponsive to treatment.

Past theories that have been proposed to account for the attacks of vertigo during the course of Meniere's disease are reviewed. In the past, vascular theories and theories of perilymph and endolymph mixing due to ruptures or leakages were proposed. Recent research concerning the basic mechanisms of the inner ear anatomy and function cast doubt on these theories. The anatomy, physiology, and pathophysiology of the inner ear, and in particular of the endolymphatic sac and endolymphatic duct are reviewed. Recent studies suggest that in people the endolymph ionic content is replenished without any flow of fluid and that longitudinal endolymph flow only occurs in response to volume excess. Furthermore audiological and electrophysiological studies have revealed little or no change in the cochlear function during episodes of vertigo. The longitudinal drainage theory attempts to encompass the recent research findings. The theory hypothesizes that endolymph draining too rapidly from the cochlear duct (pars inferior) causes attacks of vertigo. The endolymph overfills the endolymphatic sinus and overflows into the utricle (pars superior), stretching the cristae of the semicircular canals, causing the attacks of vertigo.

Some women with Meniere's disease demonstrate exacerbation of symptoms during the premenstrual period. It is believed that the hormonal stress of the premenstrual period acts on the volatile inner ear with Meniere's disease to result in dysfunction. Migraine, Meniere's disease, and the premenstrual period may be a complex interaction leading to exacerbation of symptoms. Having patients maintain a daily calendar of symptoms, diet, and menses can be helpful in understanding the disease as well as instigating treatment monitoring. Most patients can be effectively managed with dietary sodium restriction and a loop diuretic.

Meniere's disease usually begins in adults from 20 to 60 years old, and occurs in more than 10% of patients older than 65. The treatment of Meniere's disease in the elderly represents a challenge because of polymedication. Antivertiginous drugs such as betahistine and cinnarizin give good results with minor secondary effects. In contrast, major vestibular suppressor drugs such as thiethylperazin must be avoided as long-term treatment because of their side effects. Definitive vestibular surgical deafferentations such as labyrinthectomy and selective vestibular neurectomy represent optional procedures but must be carefully evaluated from case to case. Ablative procedures remain the efficient treatment of drop attacks, which represent a high potential risk of severe injuries by older patients sometimes with important social consequences.

Meniere's disease (MD), which by definition is idiopathic, has been ascribed to various causes, including inhalant and food allergies. Patients with MD report higher rates of allergy history and positive skin or in vitro tests compared with a control group of patients with other otologic diseases and to the general public. Recent immunologic studies have shown higher rates of circulating immune complexes, CD4, and other immunologic components in patients with MD compared with normal controls. Published treatment results have shown benefit from immunotherapy and/or dietary restriction for symptoms of MD in patients who present with allergy and MD.

Recent magnetic resonance imaging (MRI) techniques have made it possible to examine the compartments of the cochlea using gadolidium-chelate (GdC) as a contrast agent. As GdC loads into the perilymph space without entering the endolymph in healthy inner ears, the technique provides possibilities to visualize the different cochlear compartments and evaluate the integrity of the inner ear barriers. This critical review presents the recent advancements in the inner ear MRI technology, contrast agent application and the correlated ototoxicity study, and the uptake dynamics of GdC in the inner ear. GdC causes inflammation of the mucosa of the middle ear, but there are no reports or evidence of toxicity-related changes in vivo either in animals or in humans. Intravenously administered GdC reached the guinea pig cochlea about 10 minutes after administration and loaded the scala tympani and scala vestibuli with the peak at 60 minutes. However, the perilymphatic loading peak was 80 to 100 minutes in mice after intravenous administration of GdC. In healthy animals the scala media did not load GdC. In mice in which GdC was administered topically onto the round window, loading of the cochlea peaked at 4 hours, at which time it reached the apex. The initial portions of the organ to be filled were the basal turn of the cochlea and vestibule. In animal models with endolymphatic hydrops (EH), bulging of the Reissner's membrane was observed as deficit of GdC in the scala vestibuli. Histologically the degree of bulging correlated with the MR images. In animals with immune reaction-induced EH, MRI showed that EH could be limited to restricted regions of the inner ear, and in the same inner ear both EH and leakage of GdC into the scala media were visualized. More than 100 inner ear MRI scans have been performed to date in humans. Loading of GdC followed the pattern seen in animals, but the time frame was different. In intravenous delivery of double-dose GdC, the inner ear compartments were visualized after 4 hours. The uptake pattern of GdC in the perilymph of humans between 2 hours and 7 hours after local delivery needs to be clarified. In almost all patients with probable or suspected Meniere's disease, EH was verified. Specific algorithms with a 12-pole coil using fluid attenuation inversion recovery sequences are recommended for initial imaging in humans.

Nonoperative therapy continues to be the mainstay of treatment of patients suffering from Meniere's disease. Despite extensive research, the exact pathogenesis of Meniere's disease remains elusive. The poorly understood nature of this condition has made it nearly impossible to develop treatments that are curative. Most modern treatments are aimed at controlling symptoms. This article reviews the various nonoperative treatments that have been used to treat Meniere's disease historically as well as outlining the authors' clinical treatment paradigm.

Medical treatment for Meniere's disease is effective in controlling vertigo for approximately 85% of patients. However, when disabling vertigo continues, surgical therapy is indicated. Several surgical approaches are performed to control the symptoms of peripheral vestibular disorders refractory to medical measures, each procedure having many technical variations. Surgery is usually reserved for patients with disabling vertigo. Here, the authors discuss surgical options for vertigo control in Meniere's disease and review the literature on outcomes of these management options. The authors discuss endolymphatic sac shunt (ie, endolymphatic mastoid shunt), vestibular nerve section, cochleosacculotomy, and labyrinthectomy. When looking at data based on patient ratings, the authors find that surgery improves vertigo in endolymphatic sac shunt, vestibular nerve section, and labyrinthectomy groups and improves imbalance for the endolymphatic sac shunt and vestibular nerve section groups. Labyrinthectomy and translabyrinthine vestibular nerve section both offer excellent control of intractable vertigo. However, patients undergoing translabyrinthine vestibular nerve section are more likely to show improvement in imbalance and functional disability. This outcome is more likely for diagnoses other than Meniere's disease. There are potential prognostic factors that can be helpful in the preoperative or postoperative counseling of patients undergoing surgical treatment of vertigo. Patients who rate themselves as more disabled before surgery are less likely to achieve the best outcomes. Several other factors, such as duration of disease, contralateral tinnitus, eye disease, and allergy, may play a role.

Meniere's disease includes symptoms of fluctuating hearing loss, tinnitus, and subjective ear fullness accompanied by episodic vertigo. Along with these symptoms, patients with chronic Meniere's often develop symptoms of disequilibrium and unsteadiness that extend beyond the episodic attacks and contribute to the total disability and reduced quality of life attributed to the disease. Vestibular rehabilitation physical therapy has been used only after vestibular ablation has stabilized the vestibular loss, and for patients stably managed on medical therapy who exhibit no fluctuation in symptoms. This article reviews the data substantiating current applications of vestibular therapy, including improvements in subjective and objective balance outcome measures, and explores the possible extension of vestibular rehabilitation to treatment of patients exhibiting continued fluctuating vestibular loss.

Meniere's disease remains a disorder of unknown origin despite the collective efforts to determine the pathogenesis, although experts have long recognized that disease development likely has some heritable component. Although genetic studies of Meniere's disease have been inconclusive, increasing knowledge of human genetic structure and mutation and investigative techniques have potential to further understanding of this disorder.

FORTHCOMING ISSUES

RECENT ISSUES

THE CLINICS ARE NOW AVAILABLE ONLINE!

Access your subscription at:
www.theclinics.com

Meniere's Disease: 150 Years and Still Elusive

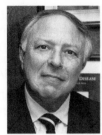 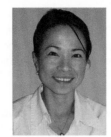

Jeffrey P. Harris, MD, PhD   Quyen T. Nguyen, MD, PhD
Guest Editors

The amount of information in the world has doubled in the past 10 years and is doubling every 18 months. Unfortunately, although nearly 150 years have passed since Prosper Ménière first described the constellation of symptoms that is called Meniere's disease, conclusive etiology and curative treatments are still elusive. Some of the brightest and most productive scientists in the world are focused on understanding the underlying mechanisms giving rise to the auditory and vestibular phenomena that patients suffer yet we still do not have a clear grasp on whether or not this disease is metabolic, developmental, genetic, autoimmune, or infectious.

Reading through the content in this publication, written by leading experts in this field, there is strong experimental and clinical evidence to support each of these theories, and thus, the most likely explanation is that the disease is multifactorial.

Although endolymphatic hydrops has long been held to be the distinguishing pathologic derangement, which gives rise to Meniere's disease, it is provocative to consider that, in blinded temporal bone studies, not all individuals with histopathologic evidence of endolymphatic hydrops had clinical histories consistent with Meniere's disease. This suggests that there may be ameliorating factors even in the presence of histopathologically evident hydrops that can modulate patient symptoms. Even more perplexing is the finding that the surgical destruction of the endolymphatic sac seems to improve symptoms in these patients, contrary to what might be expected, and calls into question the role of the endolymphatic sac in maintaining inner ear homeostasis.

Otolaryngol Clin N Am 43 (2010) xiii–xiv
doi:10.1016/j.otc.2010.05.011   **oto.theclinics.com**
0030-6665/10/$ – see front matter

Ongoing research toward the development of individualized diagnosis and thera-pies based on cellular, molecular, and genetic markers may be the key toward successful treatment of this debilitating disease and provide answers to these per-plexing observations.

Jeffrey P. Harris, MD, PhD
Chief of Otolaryngology/Head and Neck Surgery
Professor of Surgery/Otology and Neurological Surgery
University of California San Diego School of Medicine
San Diego, CA 92103, USA

Quyen T. Nguyen, MD, PhD
Department of Surgery/Otology and Neurological Surgery
University of California San Diego School of Medicine
200 West Arbor Drive, Mail Code 8895
San Diego, CA 92103, USA

E-mail addresses:
jpharris@ucsd.edu (J.P. Harris)
q1nguyen@ucsd.edu (Q.T. Nguyen)

Current Epidemiology of Meniere's Syndrome

Thomas H. Alexander, MD, MHS, Jeffrey P. Harris, MD, PhD*

KEYWORDS

• Meniere's syndrome • Prevalence • Epidemiology • Incidence

Although Meniere's syndrome (MS) has been recognized as a clinical entity for nearly 150 years since first being described by Prosper Ménière the epidemiology of the disorder is still not clearly defined. Reported prevalence rates of MS have varied widely, with estimates as low as 3.5 per 100,000 and as high as 513 per 100,000.[1–11] The wide range of values are likely due to methodological differences, changes over time in criteria for the diagnosis of MS, difficulty in distinguishing MS from related conditions such as migraine-associated vertigo,[12] and differences in the populations surveyed. The actual prevalence of MS may also be changing over time. In one report the investigators speculated that the stresses of modern society or even changes in diet have led to an increase in its occurrence over time, especially in the female population.[7]

Published reports of the epidemiology of MS generally fall into 2 methodological categories: retrospective case series and population-based surveys. Most of the studies are retrospective series that start with known cases of MS identified from patient records for a given group of hospitals and clinics. The population served by the hospitals and clinics then serves as the dominator for calculating incidence and prevalence. This methodology introduces sampling bias in that patients in the population with the disease may not have been treated at the hospitals and clinics surveyed for various reasons. Population-based cross-sectional studies reduce sampling bias by surveying a random sample of the general population. The incidence and prevalence in the general population are inferred from the exact values in the sample group. Unfortunately, for disorders such as MS that are relatively rare at the population level, very large sample sizes are needed to achieve sufficient power to accurately estimate epidemiologic characteristics in population-based studies. Radtke and colleagues[10] compared this to "searching for a needle in a haystack" with regard to MS.

Division of Otolaryngology-Head & Neck Surgery, University of California San Diego, 200 West Arbor Drive, Mail Code 8895, San Diego, CA 92103, USA
* Corresponding author.
E-mail address: jpharris@ucsd.edu

Otolaryngol Clin N Am 43 (2010) 965–970
doi:10.1016/j.otc.2010.05.001
0030-6665/10/$ – see front matter. Published by Elsevier Inc.

oto.theclinics.com

ESTIMATES OF INCIDENCE

Incidence is defined as the number of new cases occurring over a specified period of time, usually 1 year. In 1954 Cawthorne and Hewlett[1] attempted to estimate the incidence of MS by examining a register of clinical records for 8 clinical practices in Great Britain serving a population of 27,365 people; they arrived at an annual incidence of 157 per 100,000. As pointed out by Wladislavosky-Waserman and colleagues,[5] this number most likely represents a combination of incidence and prevalence, as some patients may have had onset of symptoms in preceding years.

In 1973 Stahle and colleagues[2] examined records from a standard, nationally administered records system to determine the incidence of MS in a patient population from 2 cities in Sweden; they found an annual incidence of 46 per 100,000.

Celestino and Ralli[6] reviewed the records from 1973 to 1985 from a hospital and outpatient clinic serving a community of 103,797 people in Italy. The 1972 American Academy of Ophthalmology and Otolaryngology guidelines were applied for diagnosis of MS, and an incidence of 8.2 per 100,0000 per year was found.

ESTIMATES OF PREVALENCE

Prevalence is defined as the proportion of individuals in a population having a disease. The most often-cited study examining prevalence of MS in the United States was performed by Wladislavosky-Waserman and colleagues.[5] These investigators identified cases of MS by examining medical records from 1953 to 1980 for the Mayo Clinic and Olmstead Medical Group, the major health care providers for the 40,000 inhabitants of Rochester, Minnesota. A prevalence of 218 per 100,000 in 1980 was reported. As Celestino and Ralli[6] pointed out, one-third of patients included in the Rochester study had recurrent vertigo without cochlear symptoms and would not meet current criteria for MS. Therefore, prevalence was likely overestimated. Also, the population studied was homogeneous relative to the current United States population; 99% of the subjects were white.

In 1980, Nakae and colleagues[3] reported prevalence estimates of MS based on the results of 2 nationwide surveys in Japan. The first involved a random sample of 811 hospitals and 729 clinics, and the prevalence of MS was 73 per 100,000. In the second study, all university and general hospitals in Japan (a total of 190 hospitals) were surveyed, and the prevalence was 3.5 per 100,000. It appears this number is lower than expected due to exclusion of outpatient clinics. Later surveys of more limited geographic regions in Japan, reported by Tokumasu and colleagues[4] and Watanabe,[13] yielded prevalence rates of approximately 17 per 100,000. More recently, Shojaku and colleagues[9] examined medical records from 3 hospitals in central Japan from 1980 to 2004 and found an overall prevalence of 34.5 per 100,000.

In their study of incidence of MS in Italy, Celestino and Ralli[6] calculated prevalence by multiplying the annual incidence by a conversion factor taking into account estimated life expectancy and average age of onset of MS, as previously described by Arenberg and colleagues;[14] they arrived at a prevalence 205 per 100,000.

Havia and colleagues[8] surveyed a random sample of 5000 people in Southern Finland and found a prevalence of 513 per 100,000, considerably higher than all other published results. Radtke and colleagues[10] questioned the validity of the survey used in the Havia study. These investigators suggested it may not have sufficiently discriminated vestibular from nonvestibular vertigo and did not appropriately quantify duration of attacks, leading to an overestimation of prevalence. Radtke and colleagues[10] themselves performed a survey of a random sample of 4869 people in Germany. Subjects were screened for moderate or severe dizziness or vertigo. If present, a more thorough telephone interview was performed to assess for MS using a stepwise application of the American Academy of Otolaryngology (AAO) 1995 criteria. Using this strict approach, they found a prevalence of 120 per 100,000.

To further define the current prevalence of MS in the general United States population, the authors recently analyzed data from a large health claims database containing information for over 60 million patients.[11] The database comprises fully adjudicated medical and pharmaceutical claims for over 60 million unique patients from over 97 health plans across the United States (almost 25% of the entire United States insured population). Patients in the database are representative of the national, commercially insured population on a variety of demographic measures including age, gender, health plan type, and geographic location. For the 3 years from 2005 to 2007, the prevalence among the entire United States insured population was estimated to be 190 per 100,000.

GENDER PREDOMINANCE

Reports of gender preponderance in MS have varied considerably between series. In the authors' recent United States study there was a significant female preponderance, with a female: male ratio of 1.89:1.[11] Wladislavosky-Waserman and colleagues[5] reported an overall female:male ratio of 1.57:1 (a difference they reported as not statistically significant), although they found that the incidence in women decreased significantly during each decade of the 30-year study. Early studies in Japan showed a male preponderance[13] or an equal distribution between men and women.[15] More recently Shojaku and colleagues[9] reported a 1.3:1 female:male preponderance in central Japan. Havia and colleagues[8] found a 4.3:1 female:male ratio of definite MS in their population survey in Southern Finland. These investigators felt that their rather large female preponderance was due in part to reluctance of men to participate in questionnaire studies. There appears to be some hormonal influence on MS, which may account for the gender differences.[13,16,17]

AGE OF ONSET

MS is predominantly found in adults. Reports of average age of onset range from the fourth to the seventh decades of life.[5,9,13,18] As would be expected in a chronic, nonlethal disease, the prevalence increases with increasing age. As shown in **Fig. 1**, the

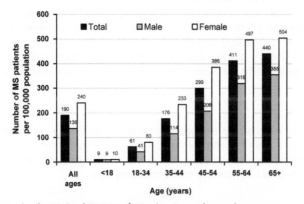

Fig. 1. Prevalence in the United States of Meniere's syndrome by age group and sex. (*From* Harris JP, Alexander TH. Current-day prevalence of Meniere's syndrome. Audiol Neurootol 2010;15(5):318–22; with permission.)

Table 1
Prevalence of selected otologic and nonotologic disorders

Condition	Prevalence per 100,000 Population	References
Meniere's syndrome (recent USA study)	190	[11]
Meniere's syndrome (previous reports)	3.5–513	[1–10]
Hearing Loss	8000–17000	[19,20]
Tinnitus	10000–15000	[21]
Vestibular vertigo (all causes)	4900	[22,23]
Benign paroxysmal positional vertigo	10–1600	[23–26]
Migrainous vertigo	890	[23,27]
Osteoarthritis	12500	[28]
Rheumatoid arthritis	600	[29]
Sjögren syndrome	186–1443	[29]
Systemic lupus erythematosus	74–150	[29]
Multiple sclerosis (in the USA)	22–160	[30]

Data from Harris JP, Alexander TH. Current-day prevalence of Meniere's syndrome. Audiol Neuro-otol 2010;15(5):318–22.

United States prevalence ranges from 9 cases per 100,000 in patients younger than 18 years to 440 per 100,000 in patients 65 years and older. Havia and colleagues[8] also reported increasing prevalence up to age 70 in Finland. The peak prevalence was 1709 per 100,000 from ages 61 to 70, with a decline to 1064 per 100,000 over age 70. Shojaku and colleagues[9] found that the incidence of MS in Japanese patients aged 65 years and older increased significantly over time from 1980 to 2004, proposing that this was a result of improved health of the elderly and an increasing population of working elderly.

COMPARISON WITH OTHER ILLNESSES

When considering the prevalence of MS, it is useful to compare it with prevalence estimates for other chronic illnesses. **Table 1** shows that MS in fact is more common than systemic lupus erythematosus and multiple sclerosis. The burden of MS in the United States is substantial, especially when considering the significant impact of MS on the quality of life of those affected. In a previous study the authors showed that MS is rated as a disorder that is disabling, significantly affects quality of life, and results in clinical depression when the disease is in its active phase.[31] Nevertheless, despite its prevalence and effect on quality of life, very few effective treatment options exist for these patients.

SUMMARY

The most recent estimate of the prevalence of MS in the United States is 190 per 100,000, a figure that is slightly lower than that reported by Wladislavosky-Waserman and colleagues[5] in 1984. MS is more likely to occur in women, and the prevalence increases dramatically with increasing age.

REFERENCES

1. Cawthorne T, Hewlett AB. Ménière's disease. Proc R Soc Med 1954;47(8):663–70.

2. Stahle J, Stahle C, Arenberg IK. Incidence of Ménière's disease. Arch Otolaryngol 1978;104(2):99–102.
3. Nakae K, Nitta H, Hattori Y, et al. [The prevalence of Ménière's disease in Japan]. Prac Otol (Kyoto) 1980;73(Suppl 2):1023–9 [in Japanese].
4. Tokumasu K, Tashiro N, Goto K, et al. [Incidence and prevalence of Ménière's disease in Sagamihara city, kanagawa-ken]. Prac Otol (Kyoto) 1982;75(Suppl 3):1165–73 [in Japanese].
5. Wladislavosky-Waserman P, Facer GW, Mokri B, et al. Ménière's disease: a 30-year epidemiologic and clinical study in Rochester, MN, 1951–1980. Laryngoscope 1984;94(8):1098–102.
6. Celestino D, Ralli G. Incidence of Ménière's disease in Italy. Am J Otol 1991;12(2):135–8.
7. Watanabe Y, Mizukoshi K, Shojaku H, et al. Epidemiological and clinical characteristics of Ménière's disease in Japan. Acta Otolaryngol Suppl 1995;519:206–10.
8. Havia M, Kentala E, Pyykko I. Prevalence of Ménière's disease in general population of Southern Finland. Otolaryngol Head Neck Surg 2005;133(5):762–8.
9. Shojaku H, Watanabe Y, Fujisaka M, et al. Epidemiologic characteristics of definite Ménière's disease in Japan. A long-term survey of Toyama and Niigata prefectures. ORL J Otorhinolaryngol Relat Spec 2005;67(5):305–9.
10. Radtke A, von Brevern M, Feldmann M, et al. Screening for Ménière's disease in the general population—the needle in the haystack. Acta Otolaryngol 2008; 128(3):272–6.
11. Harris JP, Alexander TH. Current-day prevalence of Ménière's syndrome. Audiol Neurootol 2010;15(5):318–22.
12. Radtke A, Lempert T, Gresty MA, et al. Migraine and Ménière's disease: is there a link? Neurology 2002;59(11):1700–4.
13. Watanabe I. Ménière's disease in males and females. Acta Otolaryngol 1981; 91(5–6):511–4.
14. Arenberg IK, Balkany TJ, Goldman G, et al. The incidence and prevalence of Ménière's disease—a statistical analysis of limits. Otolaryngol Clin North Am 1980;13(4):597–601.
15. Mizukoshi K, Ino H, Ishikawa K, et al. Epidemiological survey of definite cases of Ménière's disease collected by the seventeen members of the Ménière's disease research committee of Japan in 1975–1976. Adv Otorhinolaryngol 1979;25:106–11.
16. Goldman HB. [Functional recovery by endocrine treatment in Ménière's disease]. Acta Otorhinolaryngol Belg 1969;23(5):490–6 [in French].
17. Uchide K, Suzuki N, Takiguchi T, et al. The possible effect of pregnancy on Ménière's disease. ORL J Otorhinolaryngol Relat Spec 1997;59(5):292–5.
18. Yin M, Ishikawa K, Wong WH, et al. A clinical epidemiological study in 2169 patients with vertigo. Auris Nasus Larynx 2009;36(1):30–5.
19. Pleis JR, Lethbridge-Cejku M. Summary health statistics for U.S. adults: national health interview survey, 2006. Vital Health Stat 10 2007;(235):1–153.
20. Agrawal Y, Platz EA, Niparko JK. Prevalence of hearing loss and differences by demographic characteristics among US adults: data from the national health and nutrition examination survey, 1999–2004. Arch Intern Med 2008;168(14):1522–30.
21. Henry JA, Dennis KC, Schechter MA. General review of tinnitus: prevalence, mechanisms, effects, and management. J Speech Lang Hear Res 2005;48(5):1204–35.

22. Neuhauser HK, von Brevern M, Radtke A, et al. Epidemiology of vestibular vertigo: a neurotologic survey of the general population. Neurology 2005;65(6): 898–904.
23. Neuhauser HK. Epidemiology of vertigo. Curr Opin Neurol 2007;20(1):40–6.
24. Mizukoshi K, Watanabe Y, Shojaku H, et al. Epidemiological studies on benign paroxysmal positional vertigo in Japan. Acta Otolaryngol Suppl 1988;447:67–72.
25. Froehling DA, Silverstein MD, Mohr DN, et al. Benign positional vertigo: incidence and prognosis in a population-based study in Olmsted county, Minnesota. Mayo Clin Proc 1991;66(6):596–601.
26. von Brevern M, Radtke A, Lezius F, et al. Epidemiology of benign paroxysmal positional vertigo: a population based study. J Neurol Neurosurg Psychiatry 2007;78(7):710–5.
27. Neuhauser HK, Radtke A, von Brevern M, et al. Migrainous vertigo: prevalence and impact on quality of life. Neurology 2006;67(6):1028–33.
28. Lawrence RC, Felson DT, Helmick CG, et al. Estimates of the prevalence of arthritis and other rheumatic conditions in the United States. Part II. Arthritis Rheum 2008;58(1):26–35.
29. Helmick CG, Felson DT, Lawrence RC, et al. Estimates of the prevalence of arthritis and other rheumatic conditions in the United States. Part I. Arthritis Rheum 2008;58(1):15–25.
30. Pugliatti M, Sotgiu S, Rosati G. The worldwide prevalence of multiple sclerosis. Clin Neurol Neurosurg 2002;104(3):182–91.
31. Anderson JP, Harris JP. Impact of Ménière's disease on quality of life. Otol Neurotol 2001;22(6):888–94.

Endolymphatic Hydrops: Pathophysiology and Experimental Models

Alec N. Salt, PhD[a],*, Stefan K. Plontke, MD[b]

KEYWORDS

• Meniere's disease • Endolymphatic hydrops
• Ear function • Animal models

ENDOLYMPHATIC HYDROPS AND MENIERE'S DISEASE

Endolymphatic hydrops represents a pathologic anatomic finding in which the structures bounding the endolymphatic space are distended by an enlargement of endolymphatic volume. This finding was initially reported in patients with Meniere's disease by Hallpike and Cairns[1] and Yamakawa.[2] In the cochlea, endolymphatic hydrops is typically seen as a distension of the Reissner membrane into scala vestibuli (SV).[3,4] **Fig. 1** shows mid-modiolar sections through a normal and a hydropic guinea pig cochlea in which the endolymphatic compartment has been highlighted, showing the marked enlargement of the endolymphatic space and distension of the Reissner membrane. Other membranous structures in the ear may also be displaced to varying degrees, including those bounding the saccule, utricle, and ampullae of the semicircular canals.[5] The degree of distension appears to be related to the mechanical compliance of membranous components of the inner ear,[6] with high compliance (ie, mechanically weaker membranes) in the saccule and lower compliance (ie, mechanically stronger membranes) in the semicircular canals. Variations in mechanical compliance of the boundary membranes (analogous to "weak spots" on a balloon) may also explain the considerable variations in degree of hydrops in different regions of the same specimen.[7] Displacements of the basilar membrane in the apical segments of the cochlea have also been reported, in some patients to a degree whereby the basilar membrane contacts the bony wall of the scala tympani (ST).[8,9] In some specimens, membrane ruptures, herniations, and "scarring resulting from

[a] Department of Otolaryngology, Washington University School of Medicine, Box 8115, 660 South Euclid Avenue, St Louis, MO, 63110, USA
[b] Department of Otorhinolaryngology, Head and Neck Surgery, Tübingen Hearing Research Center (THRC), University of Tübingen, D-72076 Tübingen, Germany
* Corresponding author.
E-mail address: salta@ent.wustl.edu

Otolaryngol Clin N Am 43 (2010) 971–983
doi:10.1016/j.otc.2010.05.007
0030-6665/10/$ – see front matter © 2010 Elsevier Inc. All rights reserved.

oto.theclinics.com

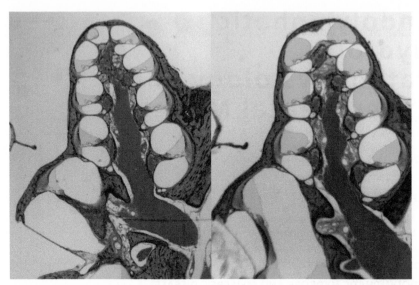

Fig. 1. Mid-modiolar sections through the normal guinea pig cochlea (*left*) and from a cochlea in which endolymphatic hydrops was induced by surgical ablation of the endolymphatic duct and sac (*right*). The endolymphatic space has been colored blue to highlight the endolymph enlargement into the perilymphatic space of scala vestibuli resulting from the distension of the Reissner membrane. Histology of these specimens was performed in the laboratory of Dr R. Kimura as part of a collaborative study (original magnification ×10).[5] (*From* Salt AN, DeMott JE, Kimura RS. Comparison of endolymph cross-sectional area measured histologically with that measured in vivo with an ionic volume marker. Ann Otol Rhinol Laryngol 1995;104:886–94; with permission.)

sealed prior ruptures" have been observed.[10] Ruptures of the boundary membranes may contribute to the episodic "attacks" and functional changes that characterize the disease.

The relationship between endolymphatic hydrops and Meniere's disease is not a simple, ideal correlation. The temporal bone specimens from patients in the early stages of Meniere's disease showed both sensory and supporting cells to be remarkably normal in appearance, hence not accounting for the functional deficits exhibited by the patient. Instead, the observation of endolymphatic hydrops in such specimens was considered as a potential cause of the disease. Careful temporal bone studies[11] have confirmed that all patients diagnosed with Meniere's disease exhibited endolymphatic hydrops in at least one ear. There were, however, a significant number (57 of the temporal bones collected from 963 patients) in which endolymphatic hydrops was observed in specimens from patients with hearing loss, albeit not necessarily fluctuating or in the low frequencies, but not exhibiting the classic symptoms of Meniere's disease; this has been termed "asymptomatic hydrops."

ANIMAL MODELS OF ENDOLYMPHATIC HYDROPS

The functional consequences of endolymphatic hydrops depend on the time course over which hydrops is induced. Acute endolymph volume manipulations are dominated by mechanical effects on the endolymphatic boundaries as they are stretched or displaced. In contrast, when hydrops develops over a prolonged period of time there are numerous additional biochemical and morphologic changes that occur. These 2 types of models of hydrops are therefore considered separately.

Acute Models of Hydrops

Injections into the endolymphatic space

The injection of an artificial endolymph into the endolymphatic system, usually into the cochlea, provides an apparently simple model of hydrops. The physiologic effects of endolymphatic injections depend on the rate and volume injected. For low injection rates, endocochlear potential (EP) is increased, due to the reduction in current through the organ of Corti as it is displaced toward ST.[12] With higher injection rates, EP decreases are observed, likely associated with chemical or mechanical trauma to the system.[13] Sirjani and colleagues[14] showed that with a low injection rate (80 nL/min) there were f_2-f_1 emission changes associated with operating point changes of the transducer and a small threshold elevation of cochlear action potential (CAP) thresholds at 2.8 kHz, whereas EP, summating potential, and CAP thresholds at 8 kHz were unchanged. With higher injection rates (200–400 nL/min) distortion and operating point changes were larger, accompanied by increases of summating potential, EP, elevations of thresholds at 2.8 and 8 kHz, and a suppression of $2f_1$-f_2 emissions. Most of these induced changes occurred transiently during the injection and recovered rapidly afterwards, a result that is not consistent with the volume injection causing a sustained hydrops. Measurements of endolymph pressure relative to that of perilymph during and following endolymphatic injections show that pressure is elevated during injections but rapidly dissipates following the injection.[6,13] Modeling the time course of pressure change during and following injection showed the pressure time course to be consistent with endolymph passing through the ductus reunions into a compartment more compliant than the cochlea (ie, the saccule).[6] Thus, the primary physiologic changes in the injection model appear to result from induced pressure changes during the injection, rather than from a sustained volume increase of cochlear endolymph. This finding contrasts with those in prolonged hydrops, as detailed later.

Cerebrospinal fluid pressure manipulations

It has been reported that in patients and animals, a decrease in hearing sensitivity may occur after leak or drainage of cerebrospinal fluid (CSF).[15–18] It has been proposed that a compensatory expansion of the endolymphatic space may be the cause of this hearing loss,[17] but this has not been proven definitively. In addition, there are case reports of large decreases in hearing sensitivity induced in Meniere's patients by manipulation of intracranial pressure,[19] but it is not known how losses are made worse by the hydropic state. Low-frequency hearing loss (without a proven hydrops) has been found in association with benign intracranial hypertension, a syndrome characterized by increased intracranial pressure without focal signs of neurologic dysfunction.[20]

Low-frequency sound

It was reported that f_2-f_1 distortion and cochlear transducer operating point changes, consistent with a displacement of the organ of Corti toward ST, were produced by low-frequency sound (200 Hz) delivered at high, but nondamaging levels (115 dB SPL).[21] Measurements of endolymph volume using a marker ion during 200 Hz, 115 dB SPL sound exposures confirmed that a substantial increase of endolymph volume (>30%) was induced by the exposure, with recovery within minutes afterwards.[22] A notable observation in this study was that in the few minutes immediately after the sound exposure, when hydrops was maximal and in the range of 20% to 30% increase relative to the normal state, cochlear sensitivity to sounds showed almost no impairment. CAP thresholds at 8, 4 and 2 kHz were all within 4 dB of the preexposure sensitivity. A contributing factor in accounting for the limited sensitivity change was an increase of EP immediately after the exposure, which would act to increase cochlear sensitivity.

Gel injection into the cochlear apex

Endolymphatic hydrops is expected to cause sustained displacements of the organ of Corti. The functional effects of a sustained displacement have been difficult to study, however, as they are technically difficult to induce. It was recently shown that slow injections of hyaluronate gel into the cochlear apex of guinea pigs produce a sustained transducer operating point change, consistent with a displacement of the organ of Corti toward ST.[23] This situation results from the resistance to the flow of gel passing through ST toward the cochlear aqueduct during injection, causing a small overpressure in SV and endolymph with respect to pressure in the basal turn of ST. In conjunction with the induced organ of Corti displacement, there was a substantial increase in EP, increases in even-order distortions ($2f_1$, f_2-f_1), decreases in odd-order distortions ($2f_1-f_2$), and decreases in cochlear sensitivity as measured by CAP thresholds. These changes were sustained throughout injections of up to 40 minutes in duration and recovered rapidly when injection stopped. In addition, following the injection of 1–2 μL of gel, the helicotrema was apparently obstructed, which produced an approximately 20 dB increase in sensitivity to stimuli of infrasonic frequencies. In the same study, a hypersensitivity to infrasound was reported in animals with surgically induced endolymphatic hydrops, presumed to result from the hydrops similarly obstructing the perilymphatic pathway between SV and ST in the apical turns. Increased sensitivity to infrasonic stimuli may account for anecdotal reports of Meniere's patients being sensitive to low frequency pressure changes, such as weather fronts and windmills.

Cyclic adenosine monophosphate manipulations

One of the earliest models for endolymphatic hydrops was the injection of cholera toxin into the endolymphatic space.[24] Subsequent studies showed that hydrops was also induced by perilymphatic administration of the toxin,[25] which was believed to act by stimulating adenylate cyclase and elevating cyclic adenosine monophosphate (cAMP). Stimulation of adenylate cyclase by forskolin was found to produce increases of endolymph Cl and of the EP.[26] An increased entry of Cl into endolymph of this model is likely to be the cause of the hydrops. In the frog, it has also been shown that ion transport was modulated by stimulation of cAMP levels with the antidiuretic hormone, vasotocin.[27]

Chronic Models of Hydrops

Surgical ablation of the endolymphatic sac

The most widely studied model of endolymphatic hydrops was created by surgical ablation of the endolymphatic duct and sac in guinea pigs.[3,4] Within a few days of sac ablation a mild hydrops developed, primarily affecting the membranes bounding the saccule, endolymphatic sinus, Reissner membrane in the cochlea and, to a lesser degree, the utricle. Initially the semicircular canals were unaffected.[3] Over the course of a few months, the hydrops became increasingly severe, with the Reissner membrane severely distended into SV and the space almost filled by endolymph after 3 to 4 months. The model was remarkable because, similar to the pathology reported at the time in Meniere's disease, it exhibited a notable endolymphatic hydrops without a major loss of hair cells or apparent damage to stria vascularis. Functional studies with this model subsequently showed that the cochlear microphonics became increasingly suppressed with time, especially for low-frequency stimuli.[28,29] Both the EP and the saccular potential decreased progressively with time.[28,30,31] This result contrasts with the cAMP-dependent models of hydrops discussed earlier, in which EP was elevated, demonstrating that the electrochemical causes/effects of endolymphatic hydrops are not consistent and vary with how the hydrops is induced. Sensitivity changes of the ear in this model, measured by CAP thresholds, were small, variable, and confined to low stimulus frequencies within the first month after surgery, progressing to become profound and affecting all frequencies after a period of 3 to 4 months.[32–34] In contrast to the enlarged summating potential (SP) reported in Meniere's patients, the increase of SP in hydropic guinea pigs was small and confined to the initial period after sac ablation,[33,35] with no SP enlargement present in the later stages when the cochlea was severely hydropic.

There are numerous histopathological changes that develop with time. In the organ of Corti of the hydropic animal, the first abnormalities are a loss of the shorter stereocilia[36] or a disarray and loss of stereocilia of the outer hair cells first occurring in the apical regions.[37] The changes at the endolymphatic surface became more severe with time and outer hair cells are subsequently lost, followed by inner hair cells, with losses greatest in the apical turns.[4,37] In the lateral wall, there are early changes in the fibrocytes of the spiral ligament.[11,38] Later intercellular edema is observed between marginal cells, an increase of vesicles, and vacuolization and atrophy of marginal and intermediate cells.[39] Changes in cellular morphology occur in the distended Reissner membrane of the hydropic cochlea. Mesothelial cells may be absent and the epithelial cells on the endolymphatic surface are enlarged,[40] suggesting the membrane has "stretched" rather than "grown." Similar changes of Reissner membrane have been observed in the hydropic human cochlea.[41] Finally, in the later stages of hydrops in both animals and humans, a loss of spiral ganglion cells occurs, primarily affecting the apical turns.[42,43]

Although initial studies suggested that endolymph Na^+ was elevated in the hydropic cochlea, several subsequent studies failed to confirm this finding. In the early stages as hydrops develops there are no significant composition changes of the major ions (K^+, Na^+, Cl^-) in either endolymph and perilymph of the hydropic ear.[28,44,45] As hydrops became more pronounced with time, a small decline in endolymph K^+, Cl^-, and osmolarity occurred in the basal turn.[44] In the normal ear, basal turn endolymph is slightly hypertonic with respect to perilymph and with respect to endolymph of the apical turns. This difference occurs even though the water permeability between endolymph and perilymph is high (equilibration half-time 7.6 minutes).[46,47] The hyperosmolarity can be accounted for by the biophysical concept of the "reflection coefficient" in which the osmotic activity of a solute depends on its permeability through the membrane dividing compartments. If the solute permeates the membrane, the osmotic pressure generated will be lower than that theoretically expected. In the cochlea, based on studies suggesting that circulating currents are carried predominantly by K^+,[48] it can be inferred that the endolymphatic boundary is more permeable to K^+ than to Na^+. If K^+ is more permeable, it will have a lower reflection coefficient, meaning that a higher concentration will be necessary in endolymph to maintain osmotic equilibrium with perilymph, for which the predominant cation is Na^+. The reduction in K^+ and osmolarity in the basal turn of the hydropic cochlea is therefore more likely related to permeability changes of the endolymphatic boundaries than to fundamental changes in ion transport processes.

In contrast to the major ions, which show only minor changes in hydrops, endolymph Ca^{2+} does show a notable increase in the hydropic ear. In the normal ear, the Ca^{2+} content of cochlear endolymph is approximately 20 μM,[49] which is extremely low relative to other extracellular fluids. In hydropic ears an increase of endolymph Ca^{2+} was observed.[50] The magnitude of the increase was subsequently found to be correlated with the decline of EP.[51] A study of EP and Ca^{2+} changes with time[31] confirmed that the Ca^{2+} increase correlated with the decline of EP as hydrops progressed. These studies confirmed that the abnormal endolymph Ca^{2+} was probably a secondary consequence of endolymphatic hydrops rather than the primary cause.[31] Nevertheless, because endolymph Ca^{2+} has been shown to influence transduction in hair cells, it is likely that endolymph Ca^{2+} changes contribute to functional losses present in the hydropic cochlea of animals, and possibly in the ears of humans with Meniere's disease too.

Aldosterone/partial sac ablation

One perceived limitation of the sac ablation model is that the endolymphatic sac is totally nonfunctional, which contrasts with the expected state for human ears with Meniere's disease. As a result there have been some attempts to induce hydrops in animals without completely ablating the endolymphatic sac. One such model used a partial dissection of the endolymphatic sac, detaching the distal portion from the sigmoid sinus while leaving the proximal, intraosseous portion undamaged. This procedure was performed in conjunction with systemic dosing of aldosterone.[52] The rationale for the use of aldosterone was based on studies showing that animals maintained on a low-Na, high-K diet developed elevated systemic aldosterone levels, which cause an elevation of Na/K ATPase levels in stria vascularis.[53] It was speculated that an enhanced secretion of K into endolymph would increase the rate of "endolymph production," which combined with partially impaired sac function could create a volume excess. The study found that aldosterone alone caused slight hydrops in some animals, while the sac dissection and sac dissection combined with aldosterone both caused moderate and severe hydrops. No details of the variations between groups were provided, so it was not apparent whether the aldosterone significantly contributed to the degree of hydrops observed. At the very least, this study demonstrates that even partial sac ablation can cause hydrops and that aldosterone may exacerbate the dysfunction.

Systemic vasopressin

It has been reported that in animals given vasopressin (also known as antidiuretic hormone, ADH) subcutaneously for 1 week by a mini-osmotic pump showed a dose-dependent increase in endolymphatic volume, with an estimated endolymph increase ratio of 17% at a dosage of 1000 U/kg/min.[54] Vasopressin (V2) receptors have been demonstrated in inner ear tissues, including the lateral wall and the endolymphatic sac,[55] and may regulate water movements through cochlear tissues by control of aquaporin expression (reviewed in Ref.[56]). By contrast, intracochlear administration of the V2 receptor antagonist OPC-31260 was shown to reverse the endolymphatic hydrops caused by endolymphatic sac ablation.[57] Ultrastructural studies show an enlargement of the intrastrial space by acutely administered vasopressin.[58] On the other hand, vasopressin plays a pivotal role in water regulation by the kidneys, being lowered at times of water excess, resulting in diuresis, and being elevated at times of dehydration to minimize urine volume. Based on the vasopressin model of hydrops, a period spent in a dehydrated state would elevate vasopressin and possibly result in the generation of endolymphatic hydrops. One study has suggested that the endolymphatic sacs of patients with Meniere's disease have significantly higher vasopressin receptor levels, suggesting that the ears of these patients may be more sensitive to vasopressin.[59] Other studies have reported elevated systemic vasopressin levels in Meniere's patients.[60–62] One recent study showed that increasing the water intake of Meniere's patients, presumed to reduce the systemic vasopressin level, reduced the severity of their symptoms.[63] While the possibility of vasopressin playing a role in endolymph volume regulation and Meniere's disease is likely, it still remains uncertain how the vasopressin/aquaporin system interacts with other hormonal systems influencing ion transport and how such a system could be controlled to achieve a stable endolymph volume in the face of varying hydration status.

Lipopolysaccharide and aldosterone

It has been reported that mice treated with intratympanic lipopolysaccharide (LPS) combined with systemic aldosterone over a 5-day period develop mild to moderate endolymphatic hydrops.[64] LPS (a toxin extracted from *Escherichia coli*) causes an immune response (a noninfectious labyrinthitis) in the ear. The advantage of this model is that it allows the endolymphatic system of the ear and of the undisturbed endolymphatic sac to be evaluated independently. Although the degree of hydrops in the cochlea was similar for LPS and aldosterone + LPS groups, the endolymphatic sac was more dilated in the aldosterone + LPS group compared with the LPS alone, in which the sac lumen was partially collapsed. A subsequent study with this model has allowed the influence of epinephrine on endolymph in the cochlea and sac to be evaluated. Epinephrine was found to increase the dilation of the intraosseous portion of the sac in the hydrops model.[65] As epinephrine has been shown to modulate K^+ secretion by marginal cells,[66] the use of this animal model allows the potential influence of different transport processes to be evaluated at the system level.

Pathophysiology of Hydrops

Pressure considerations

Both acute endolymphatic hydrops[13] and the early phase (up to 5 weeks) of chronic hydrops generally occur with negligible (<0.5 mm Hg) change in pressure between endolymph and perilymph,[67,68] because the endolymphatic boundaries are very compliant, so that endolymph volume increase can occur with very small pressure changes, less than those occurring with respiration and cardiac pulsations. For this reason it is incorrect to characterize the condition as "endolymphatic hypertension" or "glaucoma of the ear." It is generally accepted that glaucoma in the eye usually results from impaired blood flow, for which increased ocular pressure is one possible cause. Furthermore, perilymphatic pressure is not elevated in the hydropic cochlea[67–69] and is not elevated in patients with Meniere's disease,[70] so there is no perilymph pressure abnormality to influence blood flow. Even in the later stages of hydrops (>5 weeks after sac ablation), one study found no endolymph pressure increase in 33% of the animals and a mean increase of less than 1 mm Hg,[68] and another found no significant elevation at all, with a mean increase of 0.003 mm Hg.[69] These findings in the ear contrast with measurements of ocular pressure, which vary from 10 to 21 mm Hg in the normal eye and are typically greater than 22 mm Hg in patients with open-angle glaucoma. In terms of the dependence of pathology on pressure, it is apparent that endolymphatic hydrops and glaucoma of the eye are completely different and that the role pressure plays in endolymphatic hydrops is, at best, limited.

A recent study has shown that the endolymphatic sac may play some part in endolymph pressure regulation.[71] Systemic isoproterenol (β-adrenergic agonist) increased endolymph pressure and decreased the potential of the endolymphatic sac lumen, while not affecting CSF pressure. This action was suppressed in animals in which the endolymphatic sac was surgically ablated, implicating the sac as the source of the changes.

Regulation of cochlear fluids volume and composition

The relationship between ion transport and endolymph composition and volume is complex, as numerous forms of ion transport and many ion-transporting tissues bound the endolymphatic space. A disturbance of any ion transport system at any location in the ear could potentially contribute to volume disturbance. The original concept that hydrops arose due to an imbalance between endolymph secretion in the cochlea and endolymph resorption by the endolymphatic sac (impaired when the sac is ablated) has been shown to be false. Unlike many other body fluids, endolymph is not secreted in volume and does flow along the endolymphatic space at a rate that has physiologic significance.[72] The study that gave rise to the erroneous concept of endolymphatic flow[73] involved the injection of large volume of marker substance into the endolymphatic space, a procedure that has subsequently been shown to induce large nonphysiologic endolymph flows.[74] The observation that normal endolymphatic composition is maintained for days following endolymphatic sac ablation, when the hydrops is mild, further confirms that endolymph homeostasis does not require volume secretion. Instead, homeostasis appears to be dominated by the local transport of ions, with water equilibrating according to osmotic gradients, which is comparable to the situation for cytoplasm of a single cell.

Many of the ion transport processes in tissues bounding endolymph have been shown to be under the regulation of hormonal mechanisms, including β-adrenergic, muscarinic, and purinergic receptors.[66,75] The linkage between K^+ transport and endolymph K concentration and volume remains uncertain, however. Although it is commonly assumed that a change in transport of one ion (eg, K^+) will alter endolymph concentration or volume, a volume change can only occur if there is a change in transport of both K^+ and of a suitable counter ion (eg, Cl^- or HCO_3^-), allowing accumulation of electrolyte in endolymph and resulting in an osmotic influx of water. Aquaporins, also possibly under hormonal regulation, play a role in water equilibration across the endolymphatic boundaries (reviewed in Ref.[56]). So while potential elements that may be involved in endolymph volume homeostasis have been identified, it is not yet clear how these systems are integrated, and what are the specific roles of the different structures of the ear. One difficulty is the issue of how abnormal endolymph volume states are detected, given the high compliance of the endolymphatic boundaries. Pressure measurements during the initial volume injection into endolymph of the cochlea show identical pressure changes in both endolymph and perilymph, with no difference between them.[6,13] To correct abnormal volume states and to maintain the normal volume, there must be a way to detect small changes in endolymph volume status where pressure changes are minuscule. While it is accepted that the endolymphatic sac plays a primary role in endolymph volume regulation, its location (adjacent to the pulsations of the sigmoid sinus) makes it unlikely to be a sensitive mechanical detector. Furthermore, while the endolymphatic duct connects endolymph in the saccule to the sac lumen, the endolymphatic sac is not bounded by perilymph and the tissue-filled endolymphatic duct restricts the access of perilymph to the periphery of the sac. Therefore if the detection of hydrops requires the detection of a small pressure of endolymph with respect to perilymph, then the endolymphatic sac is poorly situated for this purpose. Instead, it has been proposed that the endolymphatic sinus, a small structure between the saccule and the utriculo-endolymphatic valve at the entrance to the endolymphatic duct,[76] performs this function. The walls of the sinus, similar to the membranes of the saccule, are highly distensible and their position will be sensitive to even small endolymph volume changes. It has been shown that when pressure was applied to the perilymph, the endolymphatic duct became occluded, presumably as endolymph in the sinus was displaced into the endolymphatic sac, allowing the sinus membrane to occlude the endolymphatic duct opening.[77] It is apparent that the amount of endolymph displaced from the sinus into the endolymphatic sac will depend on the degree of distension of the sinus, with more endolymph entering the sac when the sinus is enlarged. Thus the sinus could control the amount of endolymph being driven into the sac according to the volume status. The pressure fluctuations driving endolymphatic movements may include body movements (fluid inertia) or may result from tensor tympani muscle contractions, which cause the stapes to be displaced toward the labyrinth during swallowing.

Approaches to the imaging and measurement of hydrops

Endolymphatic hydrops was originally documented, and in some later studies quantified, using histologic methods that required fixation, decalcification, embedding, and sectioning of the cochlea. Several groups have quantified endolymph volume increase from scala area measurements from histologic sections either by comparison with the opposite, nonoperated ear[35] or based on the area of scala media relative to the idealized Reissner membrane position defined by a straight line between the attachment points at the spiral limbus and the lateral wall.[54,64,78] Endolymph volume in normal and hydropic cochleae was also quantified by 3-dimensional reconstructions of magnetic resonance (MR) images of fixed, but not decalcified, intact specimens.[7] One concern with all these methods is whether the degree of hydrops was influenced by the fixation and processing methods. It was shown that dissected, fresh Reissner membrane segments in vitro underwent substantial shrinkage during fixation with some protocols, suggesting that the degree of hydrops could be underestimated based on measurements from fixed tissues.[79] Recently, there have been major advances in MR imaging that have allowed endolymphatic hydrops to be visualized and quantified in the live ears of animals and humans.[80–82] These studies offer great potential to correlate the patient's symptoms or results of other diagnostic tests with the degree of hydrops as a function of time or during different therapies (eg, Ref.[82]). This subject is covered by Pyykkö and colleagues in more detail elsewhere in this issue for further exploration of this topic.

SUMMARY

Animal models of endolymphatic hydrops have provided a basic scientific understanding of endolymphatic hydrops, including the mechanical characteristics and the influence of hydrops on inner ear anatomy and function. These studies have shown that endolymphatic hydrops is accompanied by a cascade of subtle biochemical and morphologic alterations, each of which may contribute to the dysfunction. The models have allowed many hypotheses to be evaluated quantitatively, such as the possible relationships between hormonal disturbances and endolymph volume regulation. These studies have already contributed to our knowledge of endolymph physiology, and it is likely that advances from animal models will continue to contribute to the knowledge needed to control, and perhaps cure, Meniere's disease.

REFERENCES

1. Hallpike CS, Cairns HWB. Observations of the pathology of Ménière's syndrome. Proc R Soc Med 1938;31:1317–36.

2. Yamakawa K. Über die pathologische Veränderung beieinem Ménière-Kranken. Proceedings of 42nd Annual Meeting Oto-Rhino-Laryngol Soc Japan. J Otolaryngol Soc Jpn 1938;4:2310–2.

3. Kimura RS, Schuknecht HF. Membranous hydrops in the inner ear of the guinea pig after obliteration of the endolymphatic sac. Pract Otorhinolaryngol 1965;27: 343–54.

4. Kimura RS. Experimental blockage of the endolymphatic duct and sac and its effect on the inner ear of the guinea pig. Ann Otol Rhinol Laryngol 1967;76: 664–87.

5. Kimura RS. Experimental pathogenesis of hydrops. Arch Otorhinolaryngol 1976; 212:263–75.

6. Wit HP, Warmerdam TJ, Albers FW. Measurement of the mechanical compliance of the endolymphatic compartments in the guinea pig. Hear Res 2000;145:82–90.

7. Salt AN, Henson MM, Gewalt SL, et al. Detection and quantification of endolymphatic hydrops in the guinea pig cochlea by magnetic resonance microscopy. Hear Res 1995;88:79–86.

8. Nageris B, Adams JC, Merchant SN. A human temporal bone study of changes in the basilar membrane of the apical turn in endolymphatic hydrops. Am J Otol 1996;17:245–52.

9. Xenellis JE, Linthicum FH Jr, Webster P, et al. Basilar membrane displacement related to endolymphatic sac volume. Laryngoscope 2004;114:1953–9.

10. Schuknecht HF. Histopathology of Ménière's disease. In: Harris JP, editor. Ménière's disease. The Netherlands: Kugler; 1999. p. 41–52.

11. Merchant SN, Adams JC, Nadol JB Jr. Pathophysiology of Ménière's syndrome: are symptoms caused by endolymphatic hydrops? Otol Neurotol 2005;26:74–81.

12. Kakigi A, Takeda T. Effect of artificial endolymph injection into the cochlear duct on the endocochlear potential. Hear Res 1998;116:113–8.

13. Takeuchi S, Takeda T, Saito H. Pressure relationship between perilymph and endolymph associated with endolymphatic infusion. Ann Otol Rhinol Laryngol 1991;100:244–8.

14. Sirjani DB, Salt AN, Gill RM, et al. The influence of transducer operating point on distortion generation in the cochlea. J Acoust Soc Am 2004;115:1219–29.

15. Walsted A, Salomon G, Thomsen J, et al. Hearing decrease after loss of cerebrospinal fluid. A new hydrops model? Acta Otolaryngol 1991;111:468–76.

16. Walsted A, Nilsson P, Gerlif J. Cerebrospinal fluid loss and threshold changes. 2. Electrocochleographic changes of the compound action potential after CSF aspiration: an experimental study. Audiol Neurootol 1996;1:256–64.

17. Walsted A. Effects of cerebrospinal fluid loss on hearing. Acta Otolaryngol Suppl 2000;543:95–8.

18. Lee SH, Park SH, Park J, et al. Unilateral hearing loss following shunt placement for normal pressure hydrocephalus with a unilateral patent cochlear aqueduct. Clin Neurol Neurosurg 2007;109:799–802.

19. Kurzbuch AR, Momjian A, Nicoucar K, et al. Extreme sensitivity of hearing to decreases of ICP in Ménière's disease. Acta Neurochir 2009;151:1005–8.

20. Sismanis A. Otologic manifestations of benign intracranial hypertension syndrome: diagnosis and management. Laryngoscope 1987;97:1–17.

21. Kirk DL, Patuzzi RB. Transient changes in cochlear potentials and DPOAEs after low-frequency tones: the 'two-minute bounce' revisited. Hear Res 1997;112: 49–68.

22. Salt AN. Acute endolymphatic hydrops generated by exposure of the ear to nontraumatic low-frequency tones. J Assoc Res Otolaryngol 2004;5:203–14.

23. Salt AN, Brown DJ, Hartsock JJ, et al. Displacements of the organ of Corti by gel injections into the cochlear apex. Hear Res 2009;250:63–75.
24. Roheim PS, Brusilow SW. Effects of cholera toxin on cochlear endolymph production: model for endolymphatic hydrops. Proc Natl Acad Sci U S A 1976;73:1761–4.
25. Lohuis PJ, Klis SF, Klop WM, et al. Signs of endolymphatic hydrops after perilymphatic perfusion of the guinea pig cochlea with cholera toxin; a pharmacological model of acute endolymphatic hydrops. Hear Res 1999;137:103–13.
26. Kitano I, Mori N, Matsunaga T. Role of endolymphatic anion transport in forskolin-induced Cl- activity increase of scala media. Hear Res 1995;83:37–42.
27. Ferrary E, Bernard C, Friedlander G, et al. Antidiuretic hormone stimulation of adenylate cyclase in semicircular canal epithelium. Eur Arch Otorhinolaryngol 1991;248:275–8.
28. Konishi T, Salt AN, Kimura RS. Electrophysiological studies of experimentally-induced endolymphatic hydrops in guinea pigs. In: Vosteen KH, Schuknecht H, Pfaltz CR, et al, editors. Ménière's disease pathogenesis and treatment. New York: Georg Thieme Verlag; 1981. p. 47–58.
29. Kusakari J, Kobayashi T, Arakawa E, et al. Time-related changes in cochlear potentials in guinea pigs with experimentally induced endolymphatic hydrops. Acta Otolaryngol Suppl 1987;435:27–32.
30. Kusakari J, Kobayashi T, Arakawa E, et al. Saccular and cochlear endolymphatic potentials in experimentally induced endolymphatic hydrops of guinea pigs. Acta Otolaryngol 1986;101:27–33.
31. Salt AN, DeMott JD. Endolymph calcium increases with time after surgical induction of hydrops in guinea-pigs. Hear Res 1994;74:115–21.
32. Horner KC, Cazals Y. Rapidly fluctuating thresholds at the onset of experimentally-induced hydrops in the guinea pig. Hear Res 1987;26:319–25.
33. van Deelen GW, Ruding PR, Veldman JE, et al. Electrocochleographic study of experimentally induced endolymphatic hydrops. Arch Otorhinolaryngol 1987;244:167–73.
34. Horner KC. Old theme and new reflections: hearing impairment associated with endolymphatic hydrops. Hear Res 1991;52:147–56.
35. Klis SF, Buijs J, Smoorenburg GF. Quantification of the relation between electrophysiologic and morphologic changes in experimental endolymphatic hydrops. Ann Otol Rhinol Laryngol 1990;99:566–70.
36. Horner KC, Guilhaume A, Cazals Y. Atrophy of middle and short stereocilia on outer hair cells of guinea pig cochleas with experimentally induced hydrops. Hear Res 1988;32:41–8.
37. Albers FW, De Groot JC, Veldman JE, et al. Ultrastructure of the organ of Corti in experimental hydrops. Acta Otolaryngol 1988;105:281–91.
38. Ichimiya I, Adams JC, Kimura RS. Changes in immunostaining of cochleas with experimentally induced endolymphatic hydrops. Ann Otol Rhinol Laryngol 1994;103:457–68.
39. Albers FW, De Groot JC, Veldman JE, et al. Ultrastructure of the stria vascularis and Reissner's membrane in experimental hydrops. Acta Otolaryngol 1987;104:202–10.
40. Shinozaki N, Kimura RS. Scanning electron microscopic observations on the distended Reissner's and saccular membranes in the guinea pig. Acta Otolaryngol 1980;90:370–84.
41. Yoon TH, Paparella MM, Schachern PA, et al. Cellular changes in Reissner's membrane in endolymphatic hydrops. Ann Otol Rhinol Laryngol 1991;100:288–93.

42. Nadol JB Jr, Adams JC, Kim JR. Degenerative changes in the organ of Corti and lateral cochlear wall in experimental endolymphatic hydrops and human Menière's disease. Acta Otolaryngol Suppl 1995;519:47–59.

43. Bixenstine PJ, Maniglia MP, Vasanji A, et al. Spiral ganglion degeneration patterns in endolymphatic hydrops. Laryngoscope 2008;118:1217–23.

44. Sziklai I, Ferrary E, Horner KC, et al. Time-related alteration of endolymph composition in an experimental model of endolymphatic hydrops. Laryngoscope 1992;102:431–8.

45. Cohen J, Morizono T. Changes in EP and inner ear ionic concentrations in experimental endolymphatic hydrops. Acta Otolaryngol 1984;98:398–402.

46. Konishi T, Hamrick PE, Mori H. Water permeability of the endolymph-perilymph barrier in the guinea pig cochlea. Hear Res 1984;15:51–8.

47. Salt AN, DeMott JE. Endolymph volume changes during osmotic dehydration measured by two marker techniques. Hear Res 1995;90:12–23.

48. Steel KP. Perspectives: biomedicine. The benefits of recycling. Science 1999; 285:1363–4.

49. Bosher SK, Warren RL. Very low calcium content of cochlear endolymph, an extracellular fluid. Nature 1978;273:377–8.

50. Meyer zum Gottesberge AM, Ninoyu O. A new aspect in pathogenesis of experimental hydrops: role of calcium. Aviat Space Environ Med 1987;58:240–6.

51. Meyer zum Gottesberge AM. Imbalanced calcium homeostasis and endolymphatic hydrops. Acta Otolaryngol Suppl 1988;460:18–27.

52. Dunnebier EA, Segenhout JM, Wit HP, et al. Two-phase endolymphatic hydrops: a new dynamic guinea pig model. Acta Otolaryngol 1997;117:13–9.

53. ten Cate WJ, Curtis LM, Rarey KE. Effects of low-sodium, high-potassium dietary intake on cochlear lateral wall Na+, K(+)-ATPase. Eur Arch Otorhinolaryngol 1994;251:6–11.

54. Takeda T, Takeda S, Kitano H, et al. Endolymphatic hydrops induced by chronic administration of vasopressin. Hear Res 2000;140:1–6.

55. Kumagami H, Loewenheim H, Beitz E, et al. The effect of anti-diuretic hormone on the endolymphatic sac of the inner ear. Pflugers Arch 1998;436:970–5.

56. Takeda T, Taguchi D. Aquaporins as potential drug targets for Ménière's disease and its related diseases. In: Beitz E, editor, Aquaporins, handbook of experimental pharmacology, 190. Berlin (Heidelberg): Springer-Verlag; 2009. p. 171.

57. Takeda T, Sawada S, Takeda S, et al. The effects of V2 antagonist (OPC-31260) on endolymphatic hydrops. Hear Res 2003;182:9–18.

58. Nishimura M, Kakigi A, Takeda T, et al. Time course changes of vasopressin-induced enlargement of the rat intrastrial space and the effects of a vasopressin type 2 antagonist. Acta Otolaryngol 2009;129:709–15.

59. Kitahara T, Doi K, Maekawa C, et al. Ménière's attacks occur in the inner ear with excessive vasopressin type-2 receptors. J Neuroendocrinol 2008;20:1295–300.

60. Takeda T, Kakigi A, Saito H. Antidiuretic hormone (ADH) and endolymphatic hydrops. Acta Otolaryngol Suppl 1995;519:219–22.

61. Kakigi A, Takeda T. Antidiuretic hormone and osmolality in patients with Ménière's disease. ORL J Otorhinolaryngol Relat Spec 2009;71:11–3.

62. Kitahara T, Maekawa C, Kizawa K, et al. Plasma vasopressin and V2 receptor in the endolymphatic sac in patients with delayed endolymphatic hydrops. Otol Neurotol 2009;30:812–9.

63. Naganuma H, Kawahara K, Tokumasu K, et al. Water may cure patients with Ménière disease. Laryngoscope 2006;116:1455–60.

64. Takumida M, Akagi N, Anniko M. A new animal model for Ménière's disease. Acta Otolaryngol 2008;128:263–71.

65. Takumida M, Akagi N, Anniko M. Effect of inner ear blood flow changes in Ménière's model mice. Acta Otolaryngol 2009;129:244–53.
66. Wangemann P, Liu J, Shimozono M, et al. K+ secretion in strial marginal cells is stimulated via beta 1-adrenergic receptors but not via beta 2-adrenergic or vasopressin receptors. J Membr Biol 2000;175:191–202.
67. Long CH 3rd, Morizono T. Hydrostatic pressure measurements of endolymph and perilymph in a guinea pig model of endolymphatic hydrops. Otolaryngol Head Neck Surg 1987;96:83–95.
68. Böhmer A. Hydrostatic pressure in the inner ear fluid compartments and its effects on inner ear function. Acta Otolaryngol Suppl 1993;507:3–24.
69. Warmerdam TJ, Schröder FH, Wit HP, et al. Perilymphatic and endolymphatic pressures during endolymphatic hydrops. Eur Arch Otorhinolaryngol 2003;260:9–11.
70. Mateijsen DJ, Rosingh HJ, Wit HP, et al. Perilymphatic pressure measurement in patients with Ménière's disease. Eur Arch Otorhinolaryngol 2001;258:1–4.
71. Inamoto R, Miyashita T, Akiyama K, et al. Endolymphatic sac is involved in the regulation of hydrostatic pressure of cochlear endolymph. Am J Physiol Regul Integr Comp Physiol 2009;297:R1610–4.
72. Salt AN, Thalmann R. Rate of longitudinal flow of cochlear endolymph. In: Nadol JB, editor. Ménière's disease. Amsterdam: Kugler; 1989. p. 69–73.
73. Guild SR. The circulation of the endolymph. Am J Anat 1927;39:57–81.
74. Salt AN, DeMott JE. Longitudinal endolymph flow associated with acute volume increase in the cochlea. Hear Res 1997;107:29–40.
75. Wangemann P. K(+) cycling and its regulation in the cochlea and the vestibular labyrinth. Audiol Neurootol 2002;7:199–205.
76. Schuknecht HF, Belal AA. The utriculo-endolymphatic valve: its functional significance. J Laryngol Otol 1975;89:985–96.
77. Salt AN, Rask-Andersen H. Responses of the endolymphatic sac to perilymphatic manipulations: evidence for the presence of a one-way valve. Hear Res 2004; 191:90–100.
78. Salt AN, DeMott JE, Kimura RS. Comparison of endolymph cross-sectional area measured histologically with that measured in vivo with an ionic volume marker. Ann Otol Rhinol Laryngol 1995;104:886–94.
79. Brunschwig AS, Salt AN. Fixation-induced shrinkage of Reissner's membrane and its potential influence in the assessment of endolymph volume. Hear Res 1997;114:62–8.
80. Niyazov DM, Andrews JC, Strelioff D, et al. Diagnosis of endolymphatic hydrops in vivo with magnetic resonance imaging. Otol Neurotol 2001;22:813–7.
81. Nakashima T, Naganawa S, Sugiura M, et al. Visualization of endolymphatic hydrops in patients with Ménière's disease. Laryngoscope 2007;117:415–20.
82. Yamamoto M, Teranishi M, Naganawa S, et al. Relationship between the degree of endolymphatic hydrops and electrocochleography. Audiol Neurootol 2009;15: 254–60.

Physiologic Effects on the Vestibular System in Meniere's Disease

Yuri Agrawal, MD*, Lloyd B. Minor, MD

KEYWORDS

• Meniere's syndrome • Meniere's disease • Vestibular function

Meniere's syndrome is an inner ear disorder characterized by spontaneous attacks of vertigo, fluctuating low-frequency sensorineural hearing loss, aural fullness, and tinnitus. When the syndrome is idiopathic and cannot be attributed to any other cause (eg, syphilis, immune-mediated inner ear disease, surgical trauma), it is referred to as Meniere's disease.[1] Meniere's syndrome exhibits a relapsing-remitting pattern, with episodic attacks terminated by periods of restitution to normal auditory and vestibular function. In addition, the natural history of Meniere's syndrome is such that auditory and vestibular function typically decline with time.[2]

Prosper Ménière[3] first described this constellation of symptoms in 1861, and given the co-occurrence of auditory and vestibular phenomena, he proposed that the pathologic locus was the labyrinth. Subsequent investigations have corroborated his hypothesis: postmortem temporal bone analyses of individuals with Meniere's syndrome showed histopathologic abnormalities in the labyrinth. In addition, physiologic tests of labyrinthine function were also found to be abnormal in these patients. This article reviews the physiologic effects of Meniere's disease on vestibular function, as measured by caloric, head-impulse, and vestibular-evoked myogenic potential (VEMP) testing. The article begins by briefly outlining the central pathologic hypothesis behind Meniere's disease (endolymphatic hydrops) insofar as this contributes to our understanding and interpretation of vestibular physiologic tests in Meniere's disease.

ENDOLYMPHATIC HYDROPS

Endolymphatic hydrops has long been held to be the pathologic basis for Meniere's disease.[4–6] Endolymph, the potassium-enriched fluid in the inner ear, may be either excessively synthesized or inadequately resorbed, resulting in expansion of the

Department of Otolaryngology-Head and Neck Surgery, The Johns Hopkins University School of Medicine, 601 North Caroline Street, Baltimore, MD 21287, USA
* Corresponding author.
E-mail address: yagrawa1@jhmi.edu

Otolaryngol Clin N Am 43 (2010) 985–993
doi:10.1016/j.otc.2010.05.002
0030-6665/10/$ – see front matter © 2010 Elsevier Inc. All rights reserved.

endolymphatic space.[4,7] Surgical ablation of the endolymphatic sac in experimental animals has reproduced the histopathologic finding of endolymphatic hydrops seen in temporal bone specimens of individuals with Meniere's disease, although these animals do not seem to experience the classic signs and symptoms associated with Meniere's disease in humans.[8,9]

Endolymphatic hydrops typically involves the pars inferior of the labyrinth (comprising the saccule and cochlea).[6,10] Saccular hydrops may range from mild to severe, based on the degree of membrane distension toward the stapes footplate.[11] Cochlear hydrops is typified by bowing of the Reissner membrane into the scala vestibuli; severity of cochlear hydrops also varies according to the degree of convexity toward the scalar wall of the modiolus.[12] The pars superior (utricle and semicircular canals) may also be involved in endolymphatic hydrops, although changes tend to be less dramatic and occur less frequently.

Several mechanisms have been suggested to explain how endolymphatic hydrops may produce the spontaneous attacks of vertigo characteristic of Meniere's disease. The most prominent theory holds that hydropic distension of the endolymphatic duct causes rupture of the distended membranes, a phenomenon that has been observed throughout the labyrinth.[13] Membrane rupture allows the potassium-rich endolymph to leak into the perilymphatic space and contact the basal surface of the hair cells as well as the eighth cranial nerve. Initial excitation then subsequent inhibition of the hair cells manifest as a direction-changing nystagmus and may underlie the clinical phenotype of episodic vertigo.

Long-term declines in auditory and vestibular function may be the result of repeated exposure of the vestibular hair cells to toxic levels of potassium-enriched perilymph.[14] The differential susceptibility of type I and type II hair cells in Meniere's disease supports the hypothesis that chronic perilymph toxicity may cause neurosensory dysfunction.[15] The vestibular neuroepithelium consists of type I and type II hair cells as well as supporting cells. Both hair cell types have cuticular plates and stereociliary bundles, reflecting their role in mechanosensory signal transduction. However, the 2 hair cell types can be distinguished based on other morphologic characteristics: Type I hair cells are flask-shaped, have a round nucleus, and are enveloped on their basal surface by an afferent nerve chalice. In contrast, type II hair cells are cylindrical, and have oval nuclei and small bouton-type nerve terminals from afferent and efferent nerve endings.[16] The sparse nerve endings on the basal surface of type II hair cells may provide decreased protection against harmful ionic changes in the perilymph.[15] The physiologic and functional implications of the selective depletion of type II hair cells in Meniere's disease are still poorly understood.

Alternatively, it has been postulated that hydrops itself may occur in an episodic manner, as a result of sudden increases in the secretory function of the stria vascularis or of spontaneous obstruction of the endolymphatic sac.[17] Hydropic distension may then cause a mechanical deflection of the macula and crista of the otoliths and semicircular canals, respectively, and thus vestibular hair cell depolarization, leading to the sensation of vertigo.[17] Long-term changes to the neurosensory function of the vestibular apparatus may be the consequence of increased hydrodynamic pressure, causing increased vascular resistance, compromised blood flow, and chronic ischemic injury.[18,19]

Several lines of evidence challenge the primacy of endolymphatic hydrops in the pathophysiology of Meniere's disease. As mentioned previously, experimentally induced endolymphatic hydrops in animal models does not produce the clinical phenotype of Meniere's disease in these animals. Moreover, a double-blind study of temporal bone specimens and associated clinical histories reported that all individuals with Meniere's syndrome diagnosed during life had evidence of endolymphatic hydrops on postmortem examination of their temporal bones; however, not all individuals with histopathologic evidence of endolymphatic hydrops had clinical histories consistent with Meniere's disease.[20] If endolymphatic hydrops was central to the development of Meniere's disease, one would expect the correlation between the clinical manifestations of Meniere's disease and endolymphatic hydrops to be absolute.

Alternatively, studies increasingly suggest that endolymphatic hydrops may be a marker of some other pathologic process that causes Meniere's disease, such as disordered cochlear homeostasis.[21] Emerging evidence implicates the fibrocytes of the spiral ligament, which play a crucial role in maintaining cochlear fluid homeostasis; dysregulation of these cells seems to precede the development of hydrops.[22] Triggers for cytologic changes in the fibrocytes remain elusive, although this line of inquiry shows promise for yielding the true pathologic basis for Meniere's disease.

CALORIC AND HEAD IMPULSE TESTING IN MENIERE'S DISEASE

Caloric and head impulse testing are both tests of semicircular canal function. In caloric testing, bithermal irrigation is applied to the external auditory canals, which causes a convective movement of endolymph within the ipsilateral horizontal semicircular canal.[23] The movement of fluid within the horizontal canal results in excitatory or inhibitory deflection of the cupula (depending on the direction of endolymph flow). Motion of the cupula then leads to hair cell excitation or inhibition with a corresponding change in the discharge rate of vestibular-nerve afferents. Compensatory eye movements are thereby elicited (corresponding to the slow phases of nystagmus), followed by rapid corrective saccades (corresponding to the fast phase of nystagmus). The maximum velocities of the slow phases of nystagmus are compared bilaterally and used to compute unilateral weakness or caloric asymmetry. A caloric asymmetry of 20% or greater is usually considered to indicate unilateral peripheral vestibular hypofunction.

Head impulse (or head thrust) testing assesses the integrity of the three-dimensional angular vestibuloocular reflex (AVOR). Magnetic search coils are used to record head and eye movements during high-velocity, high-acceleration rotary head impulses in the plane excitatory for each of the 6 semicircular canals. Normal subjects are able to maintain visual fixation on a target during rapid head movement and thus have gain values (computed as the ratio of eye velocity to head velocity) close to 1.0.[24]

A significant reduction in the caloric response of affected ears has been observed in 42% to 79% of individuals with unilateral Meniere's disease, and caloric asymmetries of 100% (ie, absent caloric response in the affected ear) have been noted in 6% to 11% of patients.[25–31] In contrast, abnormalities of the AVOR in Meniere's disease are less prevalent. A study comparing caloric and head impulse testing in individuals with Meniere's disease observed caloric testing abnormalities in 42% of subjects but AVOR abnormalities in only 13% of patients, although a significant linear correlation was noted between head impulse test gain asymmetry and caloric unilateral weakness percentage (**Fig. 1**).[30]

The results of caloric and head impulse testing in Meniere's disease are informative. First, although caloric testing is pathologic, the normal AVOR gains in Meniere's disease suggest that there is substantial preservation of semicircular canal function in these patients.[32] In addition, although caloric and head impulse testing are measures of semicircular canal function, they seem to capture distinct phenomena. Caloric irrigation causes a slow convective flow of endolymph and provides a low-frequency stimulus to the vestibular system. In contrast, high-velocity rotary head

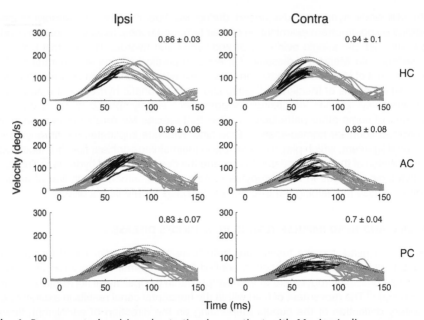

Fig. 1. Responses to head impulse testing in a patient with Meniere's disease measured before intratympanic gentamicin injection. Each panel shows head velocity (*light gray dashed*) and eye velocity (*dark gray and black*) for rotations in the excitatory direction for each canal. Data from 8 to 12 stimulus repetitions are shown for each canal. Head velocity has been inverted to permit a direct comparison of the stimulus and the response. The interval over which gain was analyzed (30 ms before peak head velocity) is shown in black for each trace. The eye velocity before and after this analysis interval is shown in dark gray. A gain value was calculated as eye/head velocity for every point in time during the analysis interval. The response gain for each stimulus repetition was defined as the maximum gain value during the interval of analysis. The response gain (mean ± standard deviation for all stimulus repetitions) is given in each panel's upper right corner. (*Reproduced from* Carey JP, Minor LB, Peng GC, et al. Changes in the three-dimensional angular vestibulo-ocular reflex following intratympanic gentamicin for Meniere's disease. J Assoc Res Otolaryngol 2002;3:430; with permission.)

thrusts cause rapid endolymph movement and generate a high-frequency input to vestibular afferents. It is possible that Meniere's disease preferentially impairs the ability of the vestibular apparatus to process low-frequency signals. The low-frequency caloric stimulus is a nonphysiologic input, whereas the high-frequency head thrust does approximate a commonly occurring stimulus. Thus it is also possible that mechanisms of central adaptation can be established only for physiologic stimuli (leading to normal responses to head impulse testing) but not for inputs outside the normal range (ie, caloric stimuli).

Further insight into the physiologic mechanisms of Meniere's disease comes from studies of the effect of chemical ablation of the peripheral vestibular apparatus using intratympanic gentamicin. Studies suggest that successful and enduring ablative therapy indicates vertigo control: patients who sustained decreases in AVOR gain and increases in caloric weakness following intratympanic gentamicin were found to have fewer episodes of posttreatment vertigo and were less likely to require repeat therapy (**Fig. 2**).[33,34] However, the correlation between the loss of semicircular

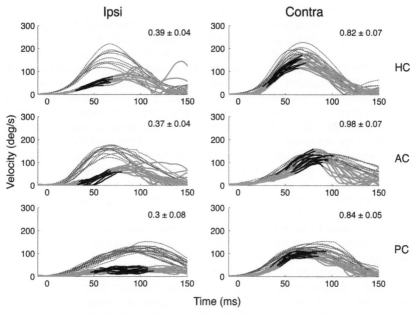

Fig. 2. Responses to head thrusts that excited each of the 6 semicircular canals in a patient with Meniere's disease (same as in Fig. 1) measured 49 days after a single intratympanic injection of gentamicin. Panels, traces, and gain values are as described for Fig. 1. (*Reproduced from* Carey JP, Minor LB, Peng GC, et al. Changes in the three-dimensional angular vestibulo-ocular reflex following intratympanic gentamicin for Meniere's disease. J Assoc Res Otolaryngol 2002;3:430; with permission.)

function and symptom control is not absolute.[34] It is possible that the natural history of Meniere's disease (typified by a high spontaneous remission rate) may obscure an association between decreased vestibular function and relief from vertigo symptoms. Alternatively, recurrent vertigo may in part reflect otolith function, which is not captured by caloric or head impulse testing.

VEMP TESTING IN MENIERE'S DISEASE

VEMPs are believed to be generated by a sacculocollic reflex. In the afferent limb of this reflex pathway, acoustically sensitive cells in the saccule respond to brief, loud, monaural sound stimuli and transmit an electrical signal centrally via the inferior vestibular nerve. The efferent limb of this reflex arc terminates in the fibers of the ipsilateral sternocleidomastoid muscle; electromyographic recordings from this muscle in response to a sound input thus reflect saccular function.[35,36] Typical VEMP testing paradigms elicit responses to broadband clicks and frequency-specific tonebursts. In normal subjects, click-evoked VEMP responses can be elicited 98% of the time and short toneburst-evoked VEMP responses occur 88% of the time.[37] Individuals with normal vestibular (ie, saccular) function also show frequency tuning of their VEMP responses, such that sound thresholds required to elicit a VEMP response are lowest when the sound stimuli are delivered at particular frequencies.[38] The greatest sensitivity of the sacculocollic reflex seems to occur in the 200- to 1000-Hz frequency range.[39,40] Frequency tuning seems to be a function of the testing apparatus as well as resonance properties of the saccule (which in part reflects the size of the saccule).

Given that Meniere's disease is associated with cochleosaccular hydrops, and that VEMP responses reflect saccular mechanics, it is logical that VEMP testing is altered in individuals with Meniere's disease. VEMP responses to click stimuli were observed to be delayed or absent in 51% to 54% of patients with Meniere's disease[41,42] compared with the normal click-evoked response rates of 98% discussed earlier. In addition, VEMP responses in individuals with Meniere's disease show altered frequency tuning, such that the greatest sensitivity of the sacculocollic reflex seems to occur at higher frequencies and across broader frequency ranges compared with normal subjects (**Fig. 3**).[43] Changes in saccular resonance characteristics in the setting of hydrops are believed to underlie the abnormalities in VEMP testing.

Further evidence that VEMP responses indicate saccular dysfunction in Meniere's disease comes from the observation of dose-response relationships. Individuals with severe saccular dysfunction who experience drop attacks (otherwise known as otolithic crises of Tumarkin[44,45]) have the greatest blunting and frequency shift of their VEMP tuning curves.[46] In addition, 27% of individuals with unilateral Meniere's disease were found to have VEMP response abnormalities in their unaffected ear; the VEMP tuning curves in these asymptomatic ears were noted to be intermediate in phenotype between affected and normal ears.[47]

VEMP testing seems to be a powerful tool in the diagnosis of Meniere's disease, likely because it specifically measures saccular function, which is impaired in Meniere's disease. A study evaluating the relative ability of various vestibular physiologic tests to predict the side of lesion in individuals with unilateral Meniere's disease found that VEMP testing using a toneburst stimulus at 250 Hz correctly assigned the side of lesion in 80% of cases.[48] This test performance was second only to the 85% correct assignment seen with caloric testing in which caloric asymmetry was defined as greater than 5% interaural difference (as opposed to the more conventional 20%–30%). Another study evaluated differences in VEMP thresholds between

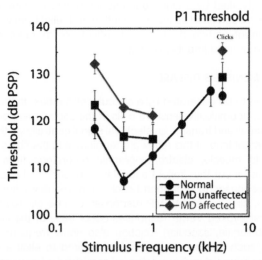

Fig. 3. Mean ± standard error of the mean VEMP thresholds for toneburst and click stimuli in ears of normal subjects (n = 14) and affected and unaffected ears of subjects with unilateral Meniere's disease (n = 34). (*Reproduced from* Rauch SD, Zhou G, Kujawa SG, et al. Vestibular evoked myogenic potentials show altered tuning in patients with Meniere's disease. Otol Neurotol 2004:25:333; with permission.)

affected and unaffected ears in patients with unilateral Meniere's disease as a measure of disease severity.[49] The investigators found a significant correlation between inter-aural VEMP amplitude differences and Meniere's disease stage based on American Academy of Otolaryngology-Head and Neck Surgery 1995 clinical criteria.[49] VEMP testing shows particular promise as a measure of Meniere's disease severity and in its ability to prognosticate bilateral disease.

SUMMARY

Cochleosaccular endolymphatic hydrops is the most consistent histopathologic finding associated with Meniere's disease. Although recent studies have questioned the etiologic role of hydrops in the pathophysiology of Meniere's disease, there is a clinicopathologic correlation that merits further characterization. Each of the vestibular tests discussed in this article (caloric, head impulse, and VEMP testing) offers unique insight into the vestibular physiology of Meniere's disease. Caloric tests seem to be the most sensitive for diagnosing Meniere's disease and determining the side of lesion in unilateral disease. Caloric testing may identify the subtle losses of vestibular function in Meniere's disease that are undetectable by other tests. VEMP testing is almost as sensitive as caloric testing, likely because it specifically measures saccular function. The threshold and frequency tuning information obtained from VEMP testing allows for a refined assessment of disease severity and can predict the onset of bilateral disease. Head impulse testing seems to be most useful at determining response to vestibular ablative therapy and associated symptom control. Head impulse testing has also shown that there is a significant preservation of vestibular function in Meniere's disease. Further understanding of vestibular physiology in Meniere's disease will be invaluable to the development of rational diagnostic and therapeutic strategies.

REFERENCES

1. Paparella MM, Sajjadi H. Endolymphatic sac enhancement. Principles of diagnosis and treatment. Am J Otol 1987;8:294.
2. Minor LB, Schessel DA, Carey JP. Ménière's disease. Curr Opin Neurol 2004;17:9.
3. Ménière P. Sur une forme de surdité grave dépendant d'une lésion de l'oreille interne. Gaz Med de Paris 1861;16:29.
4. Anatoli-Candela F. The histopathology of Ménière's disease. Acta Otolaryngol Suppl 1976;340:5.
5. Hallpike CS, Cairns H. Observations on the pathology of Ménière's syndrome. J Laryngol Otol 1938;53:625.
6. Schuknecht HF, Igarashi M. Pathophysiology of Ménière's disease. In: Pfaltz CR, editor. Controversial aspects of Ménière's disease. New York: Georg Thieme Verlag; 1986. p. 46.
7. Paparella MM. The cause (multifactorial inheritance) and pathogenesis (endolymphatic malabsorption) of Ménière's disease and its symptoms (mechanical and chemical). Acta Otolaryngol 1985;99:445.
8. Fukuda S, Keithley EM, Harris JP. The development of endolymphatic hydrops following CMV inoculation of the endolymphatic sac. Laryngoscope 1988;98:439.
9. Kimura RS. Experimental blockage of the endolymphatic duct and sac and its effect on the inner ear of the guinea pig: a study of endolymphatic hydrops. Ann Otol Rhinol Laryngol 1967;76:664.

10. Schuknecht HF. Endolymphatic hydrops: can it be controlled? Ann Otol Rhinol Laryngol 1986;95:36.
11. Horner KC. Review: morphological changes associated with endolymphatic hydrops. Scanning Microsc 1993;7:223.
12. Schuknecht HF. Pathology of the ear. Boston: Harvard University; 1974.
13. Schuknecht HF. Ménière's disease: a correlation of symptomatology and pathology. Laryngoscope 1963;73:651.
14. Thomsen J, Bretlau P. General conclusions. In: Pfaltz CR, editor. Controversial aspects of Ménière's disease. New York: Georg Thieme Verlag; 1986. p. 120.
15. Tsuji K, Velazquez-Villasenor L, Rauch SD, et al. Temporal bone studies of the human peripheral vestibular system. Ménière's disease. Ann Otol Rhinol Laryngol Suppl 2000;181:26.
16. Merchant SN, Velazquez-Villasenor L, Tsuji K, et al. Temporal bone studies of the human peripheral vestibular system. Normative vestibular hair cell data. Ann Otol Rhinol Laryngol Suppl 2000;181:3.
17. Honrubia V. Pathophysiology of Ménière's disease: vestibular system. In: Harris JP, editor. Ménière's disease. The Hague: Kugler Publications; 1999. p. 231.
18. Andrews JC, Honrubia V. Vestibular function in experimental endolymphatic hydrops. Laryngoscope 1988;98:479.
19. Nakashima T, Ito A. Effect of increased perilymphatic pressure on endocochlear potential. Ann Otol Rhinol Laryngol 1981;90:264.
20. Rauch SD, Merchant SN, Thedinger BA. Ménière's syndrome and endolymphatic hydrops. Double-blind temporal bone study. Ann Otol Rhinol Laryngol 1989;98:873.
21. Merchant SN, Adams JC, Nadol JB Jr. Pathophysiology of Ménière's syndrome: are symptoms caused by endolymphatic hydrops? Otol Neurotol 2005;26:74.
22. Shinomori Y, Kimura RS, Adams JC. Changes in immunostaining for Na+, K+, 2Cl-cotransporter 1, taurine and c-Jun N-terminal kinase in experimentally induced endolymphatic hydrops. ARO Abstr 2001;24:134.
23. Proctor L, Dix R, Hughes D, et al. Stimulation of the vestibular receptor by means of step temperature changes during continuous aural irrigation. Acta Otolaryngol 1975;79:425.
24. Aw ST, Haslwanter T, Halmagyi GM, et al. Three-dimensional vector analysis of the human vestibuloocular reflex in response to high-acceleration head rotations. I. Responses in normal subjects. J Neurophysiol 1996;76:4009.
25. Black FO, Kitch R. A review of vestibular test results in Ménière's disease. Otolaryngol Clin North Am 1980;13:631.
26. Enander A, Stahle J. Hearing loss and caloric response in Ménière's disease. A comparative study. Acta Otolaryngol 1969;67:57.
27. Hone SW, Nedzelski J, Chen J. Does intratympanic gentamicin treatment for Ménière's disease cause complete vestibular ablation? J Otolaryngol 2000;29:83.
28. Martin E, Perez N. Hearing loss after intratympanic gentamicin therapy for unilateral Ménière's Disease. Otol Neurotol 2003;24:800.
29. Oosterveld WJ. Ménière's disease, signs and symptoms. J Laryngol Otol 1980; 94:885.
30. Park HJ, Migliaccio AA, Della Santina CC, et al. Search-coil head-thrust and caloric tests in Ménière's disease. Acta Otolaryngol 2005;125:852.
31. Stahle J, Klockhoff I. Diagnostic procedures, differential diagnosis and general conclusions. In: Pfaltz CR, editor. Controversial aspects of Ménière's disease. New York: Georg Thieme Verlag Stuttgart; 1986. p. 71.

32. Carey JP, Minor LB, Peng GC, et al. Changes in the three-dimensional angular vestibulo-ocular reflex following intratympanic gentamicin for Ménière's disease. J Assoc Res Otolaryngol 2002;3:430.

33. Lin FR, Migliaccio AA, Haslwanter T, et al. Angular vestibulo-ocular reflex gains correlate with vertigo control after intratympanic gentamicin treatment for Ménière's disease. Ann Otol Rhinol Laryngol 2005;114:777.

34. Nguyen KD, Minor LB, Della Santina CC, et al. Vestibular function and vertigo control after intratympanic gentamicin for Ménière's disease. Audiol Neurootol 2009;14:361.

35. Colebatch JG, Halmagyi GM. Vestibular evoked potentials in human neck muscles before and after unilateral vestibular deafferentation. Neurology 1992; 42:1635.

36. McCue MP, Guinan JJ Jr. Acoustically responsive fibers in the vestibular nerve of the cat. J Neurosci 1994;14:6058.

37. Cheng PW, Huang TW, Young YH. The influence of clicks versus short tone bursts on the vestibular evoked myogenic potentials. Ear Hear 2003;24:195.

38. Cheng PW, Murofushi T. The effects of plateau time on vestibular-evoked myogenic potentials triggered by tone bursts. Acta Otolaryngol 2001;121:935.

39. Todd NP, Cody FW, Banks JR. A saccular origin of frequency tuning in myogenic vestibular evoked potentials? Implications for human responses to loud sounds. Hear Res 2000;141:180.

40. Welgampola MS, Colebatch JG. Characteristics of tone burst-evoked myogenic potentials in the sternocleidomastoid muscles. Otol Neurotol 2001;22:796.

41. de Waele C, Huy PT, Diard JP, et al. Saccular dysfunction in Ménière's disease. Am J Otol 1999;20:223.

42. Murofushi T, Shimizu K, Takegoshi H, et al. Diagnostic value of prolonged latencies in the vestibular evoked myogenic potential. Arch Otolaryngol Head Neck Surg 2001;127:1069.

43. Rauch SD, Zhou G, Kujawa SG, et al. Vestibular evoked myogenic potentials show altered tuning in patients with Ménière's disease. Otol Neurotol 2004; 25:333.

44. Baloh RW, Jacobson K, Winder T. Drop attacks with Ménière's syndrome. Ann Neurol 1990;28:384.

45. Tumarkin A. The otolithic catastrophe: a new syndrome. BMJ 1936;2:175.

46. Timmer FC, Zhou G, Guinan JJ, et al. Vestibular evoked myogenic potential (VEMP) in patients with Ménière's disease with drop attacks. Laryngoscope 2006;116:776.

47. Lin MY, Timmer FC, Oriel BS, et al. Vestibular evoked myogenic potentials (VEMP) can detect asymptomatic saccular hydrops. Laryngoscope 2006;116:987.

48. Rauch SD, Silveira MB, Zhou G, et al. Vestibular evoked myogenic potentials versus vestibular test battery in patients with Ménière's disease. Otol Neurotol 2004;25:981.

49. Young YH, Huang TW, Cheng PW. Assessing the stage of Ménière's disease using vestibular evoked myogenic potentials. Arch Otolaryngol Head Neck Surg 2003;129:815.

Audiovestibular Testing in Patients with Meniere's Disease

Meredith E. Adams, MD[a], Katherine D. Heidenreich, MD[b],
Paul R. Kileny, PhD[b],*

KEYWORDS

• Meniere's disease • Audiovestibular testing • VEMP testing
• ECoG testing

One hundred and fifty years after Prosper Ménière[1] described the symptom complex of recurring episodic vertigo, hearing loss, and tinnitus, the diagnosis of Meniere's disease (MD) remains challenging for the clinician. In part, we are limited by the confines of inner ear diagnostics. Postmortem histopathologic examinations of human temporal bones have shown that many patients with classic MD have distortion and dilation of the endolymphatic spaces of the membranous labyrinth, a finding known as endolymphatic hydrops.[2] These alterations are proposed to be the pathologic basis of MD; however, the correlation between these histologic changes and the clinical manifestations of MD is not absolute. For example, in a double-blind temporal bone study, Rauch and colleagues[2] found histologic evidence of endolymphatic hydrops in 13 of 13 cases of clinical MD, but review of medical records of 6 of 19 temporal bones with endolymphatic hydrops did not reveal symptoms or signs of MD.[3] Thus, many inner ears may have hydropic changes without manifesting the clinical syndrome. Some have suggested that endolymphatic hydrops may be an epiphenomenon of the true, as yet undiscovered, pathophysiologic mechanism of MD.[4]

Without definitive diagnostic criteria for MD, clinicians must rely on historical information and other clinical features to make the diagnosis. At present, by the American Academy of Otolaryngology–Head & Neck Surgery (AAO–HNS) criteria, the diagnosis of MD depends on symptoms of recurrent, spontaneous vertigo, hearing loss, aural fullness, and tinnitus, as well as objective documentation of hearing loss, with other potential causes excluded by proper otologic investigation.[5] The presence and

[a] Department of Otolaryngology-Head and Neck Surgery, University of Minnesota, 420 Delaware Street SE, Minneapolis, MN 55455, USA
[b] Department of Otolaryngology-Head and Neck Surgery, University of Michigan Health System, 1904 Taubman Center, 1500 East Medical Center Drive, SPC 5312, Ann Arbor, MI 48109-5312, USA
* Corresponding author.
E-mail address: pkileny@umich.edu

Otolaryngol Clin N Am 43 (2010) 995–1009
doi:10.1016/j.otc.2010.05.008
0030-6665/10/$ – see front matter © 2010 Elsevier Inc. All rights reserved.

oto.theclinics.com

severity of symptoms may fluctuate frequently over time, and physical findings are generally lacking. Thus, there continues to be a strong interest in identifying additional means of testing for MD.

In this article, the present state of the art with respect to audiovestibular testing for MD is reviewed. Because there is no gold standard for MD diagnosis, it is impossible to measure the performance characteristics of the various test methods. The classic dictum is that even the "best" tests yield positive results in only two-thirds of patients with classic MD. Still, we advocate the use and further investigation of advanced audiovestibular testing in patients with MD in an attempt to answer several questions confronting any clinician who cares for patients with audiovestibular symptoms:

1. Does the patient have MD? We review how audiometry can be used to determine if a patient fulfills the AAO–HNS criteria for MD.[5] Audiovestibular testing is also particularly useful for patients who present with only portions of the classic symptom complex. In such cases, objective testing might differentiate a patient likely to have MD with normal hearing at baseline from one with migraine-associated vertigo. Tests may also detect incipient MD, allowing us to initiate nondestructive treatments at earlier stages.
2. Which ear is causing the symptoms? Audiovestibular testing can be used to simplify difficult treatment decisions. If we are able to confirm the diagnosis and lateralize the pathology to one ear, we can proceed with potentially destructive therapy with more confidence.
3. Is there bilateral disease now, or might there be in the future? It is estimated that 30% of patients with MD will develop bilateral disease.[6-8] It would be helpful to be able to exclude or confirm contralateral disease when considering the treatment approach for the first ear.
4. Is our treatment effective? Once therapy is initiated, it would be desirable to monitor the patient for progression or remission. Expansion of the knowledge of the available and emerging investigative methods may facilitate critical evaluation of treatment regimens and interventions targeted at halting disease progression.

AUDIOMETRIC TESTING

Hearing loss in patients with MD is predominantly sensorineural, fluctuating, and progressive. The hearing loss tends to involve the low frequencies early in the course of the disease. Higher frequencies may also be affected, and some have observed a peak, or inverted-V, audiogram in patients with MD.[9] With time, the hearing loss tends to flatten and become less variable.[10] Nevertheless, there is no audiometric configuration that can be considered characteristic of MD, and the configuration does not depend on disease duration.[10,11] Fluctuation of pure tone thresholds, word recognition, or both is commonly noted. In patients with long-standing MD (>10 years), the average pure tone threshold in the affected ear stabilizes at about 50 dB, and the mean word recognition score reaches a minimum of 50%.[10] Profound hearing loss occurs in only 1% to 2% of patients.[12] The sensorineural hearing loss is cochlear in etiology, with associated distortion, loudness recruitment, and a reduction of word recognition scores in proportion to the pure tone average.

It is interesting to note that a mild low-frequency conductive hearing loss is not uncommonly observed early in the course of the disease. Muchnik and colleagues[13] observed a low-frequency air-bone gap with no middle ear pathology and normal acoustic reflexes in 33% (13 of 40) of patients with classic MD. Although some have dismissed this finding as artifactual, it is reasonable to propose that this is an "inner ear conductive hearing loss," as a result of increased inner ear fluid volume and pressure (related to endolymphatic hydrops) dampening the stapes footplate mobility.[13] In retrospect, these studies may have included some patients with vestibular symptoms and low-frequency conductive hearing loss secondary to undetected superior semicircular canal dehiscence. The clinician should keep this entity in mind when confronted with such a presentation.

AAO–HNS Guidelines

As defined by the 1995 AAO–HNS Committee on Hearing and Equilibrium, diagnostic guidelines for MD require defined historical criteria (vertigo, tinnitus, aural fullness) and audiometrical documentation of sensorineural hearing loss in the suspect ear on at least one occasion. The hearing loss may take any of the following forms: (1) average thresholds at 250, 500, and 1000 Hz at least 15 dB higher than the average of 1, 2, and 3 kHz; (2) in unilateral cases, the 4-frequency pure tone average of thresholds at 0.5, 1.0, 2.0, and 3.0 kHz is at least 20 dB poorer in the affected ear than in the contralateral ear; (3) in bilateral cases, the 4-frequency pure tone average is greater than 25 dB in the studied ear; or (4) the clinician judges that the patient's hearing loss meets reasonable audiometric criteria for hearing loss characteristic of MD. A change of 10 dB in the 4-tone average or of 15% in word recognition score is considered clinically significant fluctuation.[5] To avoid the subjectivity and ambiguity inherent in a staging system based on hearing, vestibular, and other symptoms, the Committee also proposed a staging system based solely on hearing as measured by audiometry. All patients will not progress through all stages in sequence, but this system may aid in the analysis of treatment results. The stages are based on the 4-frequency pure tone average, in dB, of the worst audiogram during the 6-month interval before treatment, as follows: (1) 25 or less, (2) 26 to 40, (3) 41 to 70, (4) greater than 70.[5]

Loudness Recruitment

To support a diagnosis of MD, some clinician-investigators have exploited the psychoacoustic phenomenon of loudness recruitment, defined as the abnormal growth of perceived loudness with increasing stimulus intensity. In a series of 200 patients with clinical features of MD, all were found to have recruitment, regardless of the severity of their hearing loss.[14] The most straightforward test of loudness recruitment is the alternate binaural loudness balance test (ABLB). In this procedure, auditory stimuli are presented to both ears, and the stimulus intensity in the suspect ear is adjusted until its perceived loudness is equal to that in the other ear. These results are then plotted as a function of healthy ear stimulus intensity (ie, with the suspect-ear threshold on the x-axis and the other ear threshold on the y-axis). Recruitment is evidenced by a slope function greater than 1. This test is time-consuming and can be challenging for some patients. We do not routinely use the ABLB at our institution, but we often look for indirect evidence of recruitment by history and audiometry (eg, complaints of sound sensitivity in the affected ear, decreased most-comfortable loudness level, narrowed dynamic range, or elicitation of an acoustic reflex at a level that would typically be subthreshold in a normal ear). Although commonly associated with endolymphatic hydrops, recruitment is present in numerous nonhydropic etiologies of cochlear hearing loss, and is therefore not specific for MD.

VESTIBULAR TESTING

Vestibular test results are not included in the 1995 AAO–HNS Guidelines for the Diagnosis and Evaluation of Therapy in MD, and, strictly speaking, are not necessary for the diagnosis of MD. Although the audiogram remains the most widely used clinical test for MD, it is the vertigo attacks that are often the most disabling symptom of the disease. There is no reason to insist that audiometric changes will directly correlate with vestibular symptoms. Thus, some physicians have argued that vestibular tests can be a useful adjunct in identifying the diseased ear(s) in patients with MD whose symptoms and audiogram are nonlateralizing, and for monitoring the development of early disease in the contralateral ear.[15,16] Use of vestibular testing in the evaluation of patients with MD remains controversial, however, as these test results often fluctuate during the course of the disease, cannot reliably identify the affected ear, and the degree of damage detected correlates poorly with patient-perceived disability. Currently, the most widespread application of vestibular testing in MD has been to exclude pathology in the contralateral labyrinth in patients who are candidates for ablative therapy.

Caloric Testing

Caloric testing represents a nonphysiologic, low-frequency (~ 0.003 Hz) stimulation of the horizontal semicircular canal. It is the only test in the standard vestibular test battery that provides lateralizing information. The definition of a clinically significant caloric asymmetry varies from laboratory to laboratory, but most institutions consider a 20% to 28% or greater canal paresis by Jongkee's formula to be abnormal. This common vestibular test abnormality is reported in up to 50% to 66% of MD patients.[17,18] This leaves a significant proportion of patients with MD who will have no evidence of pathology on caloric testing. Furthermore, there does not appear to be a clear relationship between the development of canal paresis and duration of symptoms in the ear with MD.[19,20] The magnitude of caloric paresis ranges from 25% to 50%, and complete loss of caloric response is rare.[21,22] Based on temporal bone studies, the mechanism for caloric paresis in MD may be related to ampullary distortion with disruption of the attachment of the cupula.[23]

Use of caloric data to identify the affected ear in MD is highly controversial. Dimitri and colleagues[15] argued that if a 5% interaural caloric difference was used in a forced choice paradigm, this test could correctly identify the diseased ear in 95% of cases; however, most institutions continue to use Jongkee's formula as a benchmark for pathologic asymmetry. Using these more widely accepted criteria, canal paresis has been documented in the *contralateral* ear in up to 19% of patients with unilateral MD who underwent serial vestibular testing,[22] which may represent an irritative lesion.

Caloric data are often considered essential before administering any form of ablative therapy in unilateral MD to confirm that the contralateral labyrinth is functional. Complete loss of vestibular function as manifested by absent caloric response to ice water irrigation need not be pursued as a therapeutic end point in intratympanic gentamicin therapy, as it is not required for vertigo control in MD, and is associated with an unacceptably high rate of sensorineural hearing loss in the treated ear.[24,25]

Spontaneous Nystagmus

The second most common abnormality seen during videonystagmography in patients with MD is spontaneous nystagmus. It is often seen during an acute attack or within days following an attack. Three larger series found that spontaneous nystagmus was present in 20% to 67% of patients with MD, but there is a lack of consensus regarding the criteria for pathologic spontaneous nystagmus.[22,26,27] The direction of the observed spontaneous nystagmus varies; it can consistently beat toward the involved ear (irritative), away from it (paralytic), or change from an irritative to a paralytic pattern over time, and thus cannot be used to lateralize the disease. Some authors have attempted to explain the irritative pattern of nystagmus with the membrane rupture theory, arguing that ruptures of inner ear membranes allow the potassium-rich endolymph to transiently leak into the perilymph that bathes the VIIIth nerve and basal surfaces of the hair cells. The resultant potassium intoxication leads to an initial partial depolarization of the vestibular nerve with an increase in the resting discharge rate (irritative lesion). This may then be followed by complete depolarization and inhibition from a blockade of transmitter release (paralytic lesion).[3,28]

Spontaneous nystagmus can be a useful clinical finding when following patients with MD who undergo intratympanic gentamicin therapy. Minor[25] found that development of spontaneous nystagmus beating away from the treated ear was 1 of 3 clinical signs that specified completion of intratympanic gentamicin therapy, and was associated with a high vertigo control rate. This does not require formal videonystagmography and can be easily done at the bedside with Frenzel lenses.

Rotational Testing

Rotational testing is a natural stimulus for the peripheral vestibular system and relies on angular acceleration. It assesses more physiologically relevant frequencies of the vestibulo-ocular reflex (VOR) compared with caloric testing. It is nonlateralizing. The 2 most common methods to rotate a patient are (1) passive rotation of the head and body in the horizontal plane with rotary chair, or (2) autorotation. This latter method uses active head rotation and can be used in either the horizontal or vertical planes.

Rotary chair test findings in MD are extremely nonspecific and various abnormalities have been described in a small number of studies. Palomar-Asenjo and colleagues[26] found that 23% of patients with MD had elevated phase leads in at least 2 consecutive frequencies on sinusoidal harmonic acceleration. Decreased, normal, and elevated gains have been described in patients with MD.[21,26] Autorotation may permit assessment of higher VOR frequencies compared with rotary chair, but its test-retest reliability is unclear.[29]

Posturography

Computerized dynamic posturography (CDP) tests postural control in 6 different conditions designed to emphasize or minimize vestibular, visual, and proprioceptive input. It provides useful information about a patient's functional balance status, but does not directly assess deficits in any of these 3 sensory systems. There is some interest in use of posturography in MD to stage the degree of functional impairment.[30]

VESTIBULAR EVOKED MYOGENIC POTENTIALS

Vestibular evoked myogenic potential (VEMP) testing is a more recent addition to the MD diagnostic armamentarium. The VEMP is obtained by measuring the relaxation of the sternocleidomastoid muscle (SCM) in response to an ipsilateral auditory stimulus. Brief high-intensity monaural clicks or tone-bursts produce a large, short-latency inhibitory potential (VEMP) in the tonically contracted ipsilateral SCM.[31] Although the exact neural pathway is still not fully clear, the VEMP is considered to be a vestibulocollic reflex with the afferent limb arising from sound-responsive sensory cells in the saccule. The afferent signal is conducted centrally via the inferior vestibular nerve, and efferent signal is conducted via the vestibulo-spinal track to produce inhibitory postsynaptic potentials in cervical motor neurons.[32,33] Normal responses are composed of biphasic (positive-negative) waves. By convention, they are labeled "p" (for positive) and "n" (for negative), followed by their mean latency value in milliseconds.[32] The first wave complex, present in most healthy participants, is labeled p13-n23.

VEMP testing is a useful adjunct to other studies because it can reveal saccule dysfunction. After the cochlea, the saccule is the second most common site of hydropic changes in temporal bones of patients with MD.[34] It is reasonable to expect that the altered mechanics of a distended saccule might lead to an altered VEMP in MD.[35] This hypothesis has been verified by several studies. Although Cheng and colleagues[36] detected click-evoked VEMP (C-VEMPs) in 98% of normal ears, De Waele and colleagues[37] reported that C-VEMPs were absent in 54% of patients with MD. In another retrospective review, Murofushi and colleagues[38] found that the C-VEMP response was significantly reduced in amplitude or absent in 51% of patients with MD.

Rauch and others[35,38,39] have suggested that the diagnostic utility of VEMP may be improved using threshold measures for tone burst stimuli (TB-VEMP). Healthy adults have frequency-dependent TB-VEMP thresholds, with the best response occurring at 500 Hz. In practical terms, a patient has normal frequency tuning if the threshold for a 500-Hz TB-VEMP is less than the thresholds for 250-Hz and 1000-Hz stimuli. In their prospective cohort study of 14 healthy adults and 34 adults with unilateral MD by AAO–HNS criteria, Rauch and colleagues[35] observed that the affected ears of patients with MD had significantly increased TB-VEMP thresholds compared with unaffected ears and healthy subjects. Furthermore, affected ears demonstrated alterations in frequency-tuning (eg, threshold at 500 Hz >at 1000 Hz), and the VEMP threshold did not correlate with ipsilateral audiometric thresholds. Interestingly, the "Meniere's-like" response was also observed in the unaffected ears of some patients with MD.[35] In a follow-up study, Lin and colleagues[40] found that 27% of patients with unilateral MD showed elevated thresholds and altered tuning characteristics in the asymptomatic ear. This is similar to the 30% rate of second ear involvement reported in the literature, and to the 35% rate of occult saccular hydrops in the asymptomatic ear discovered in their concurrent review of postmortem temporal bones from patients with unilateral MD. They propose that VEMP may be used not only as an adjunct to predict the side of disease,[41] but also as a potential clinical detector of "presymptomatic" hydrops, and thus may be used to predict the development of bilateral disease.[40] Prospective clinical trials are under way in this regard.

ELECTROCOCHLEOGRAPHY

Electrocochleography (ECoG) is the measurement of the electrical potentials generated by the cochlea and the auditory nerve in response to acoustic stimulation. The technique is similar to ABR measurement, in that an auditory stimulus is presented to the test ear and an electrical response is recorded. In the case of ABR, the recording electrode is placed on the scalp, and the response of the auditory nerve and brainstem is measured. The pertinent time epoch consists of the first 10 ms after stimulus presentation. In the case of ECoG, the recording electrode is placed as close to the cochlea as possible (near-field recording), and the response of interest is measured from the cochlear hair cells and auditory nerve. The epoch of interest is generally within the first 3 ms following stimulus presentation.

Depending on the nature of the stimulus and the mode of stimulus delivery, the ECoG response may consist of a combination of the *cochlear microphonic* (CM), the *summating potential* (SP), and cochlear nerve compound *action potential* (AP). The CM is an alternating current (AC) potential, closely resembling the stimulus, which is generated mainly by outer hair cells (OHCs),[42] and generally reflects activity in OHCs closest to the recording electrode (eg, the basal portion of the basilar membrane for extracochlear recording). The CM parallels the waveform of the stimulus and the vibrations of the basilar membrane (hence the term, *microphonic*), so if the polarity of the stimulus is reversed (eg, from condensation to rarefaction), the polarity of the CM reverses. The CM is present as long as the stimulus is presented, so alternate polarity stimuli are used to effectively reduce (or cancel) the amplitude of the CM so that the next ECoG components may be measured. A normal cochlear microphonic response is shown in the upper tracing of **Fig. 1**. The SP is a direct current (DC) potential, and consists of a shift in the baseline of a CM. When a brief constant-polarity tone-burst is the stimulus, the SP will appear as a shift in the baseline of the CM (or a "pedestal" carrying the CM). When the stimulus is a click alternated in polarity, the SP will appear as a deflection preceding the onset of the AP, with the same polarity. The SP appears as a DC potential, and its duration is that of the stimulus. Although inner hair cells (IHCs) are particularly important in the production of the SP, there is also a significant contribution from OHCs.[43] The AP is the sum of the individual action potentials of synchronously firing auditory nerve fibers, and is equivalent to wave I of the ABR. The polarities of the SP and AP measured at the tympanic membrane or promontory are usually the same, and are independent of the polarity of the stimulus. Whether the SP and/or the AP have a positive or negative polarity in a given recording depends on the connection of the recording and reference electrodes (*anode* or *cathode*).

ECoG can be performed with click or tone-burst stimuli. With click stimuli, the amplitude of the SP is most easily obtained by presenting a train of alternating condensation and rarefaction clicks or by obtaining the sum of condensation and rarefaction stimulation. By using alternating polarity, the CM response is averaged out (ie, cancelled) and the SP is seen as a "knee" preceding the up-slope of the AP waveform. **Fig. 2** illustrates an electrocochleographic response elicited by an alternating click presented at 85-dB nHL and clearly consists of a well-defined SP and AP. With a tone-burst stimulus duration of several milliseconds, the amplitude of the CM is measured from the peak-to-peak amplitude during the stable portion of the response. To measure the SP, one must account for the baseline shift that occurs from the prestimulus to the poststimulus interval. The SP amplitude is measured from the "moving baseline" drawn from the prestimulus and poststimulus response to the midpoint of

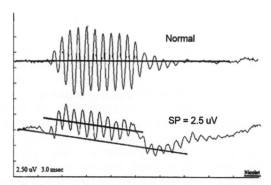

Fig. 1. Tympanic membrane recordings of ECoG responses to 1-kHz tone bursts. The upper trace represents a pure CM response with no discernable SP component. The lower trace illustrates the CM superimposed on an elevated SP in a patient with Meniere's disease. The CM amplitude is measured peak to peak at the widest point. The SP amplitude is calculated by first determining a "moving baseline" by connecting the prestimulus baseline to the poststimulus baseline, as shown. The SP is the difference between the moving baseline and the midpoint of the peak-to-peak CM waveform.

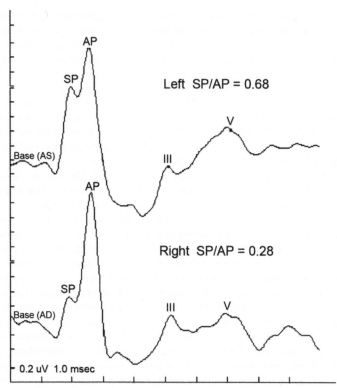

Fig. 2. Click-evoked ECoG response recorded with a hydrogel tympanic membrane surface electrode in a patient with Meniere's disease in the left ear. This response was elicited by an alternating click stimulus presented at 85 dB nHL. The SP and AP are measured from the prestimulus baseline. Note the increased SP in the diseased left ear. SP, summating potential; AP, cochlear nerve action potential.

the peak-to-peak CM response at its greatest distance from the baseline. An example of this in a patient with MD is shown in the lower trace of **Fig. 1**.

Optimally, the measurement of these potentials is performed with an electrode placed as close as possible to their source to maximize response amplitude. Such near-field recording can be performed with a silver ball electrode placed on the round window membrane. Because this requires surgical exposure of the middle ear, it is not widely accepted for routine outpatient clinical applications. An alternative method is the use of a transtympanic promontory needle electrode referenced to an electrode external to the ear (forehead or tragus). Less invasive recording may be performed with electrodes placed in the external ear canal or on the surface of the tympanic membrane. The latter is gaining in popularity because of ease of placement and the clarity and amplitude of the responses it provides. One type of tympanic membrane (TM) surface electrode consists of a soft, hydrogel tip encasing a silver wire threaded through a soft polyethylene tube. This electrode is positioned gently onto the central portion of the lateral surface of the TM under microscopic visualization (**Fig. 3**). Although the amplitude of the response obtained with the tympanic membrane surface electrode is attenuated compared with a transtympanic needle recording, its ease of placement, patient comfort, and noninvasive nature outweigh this

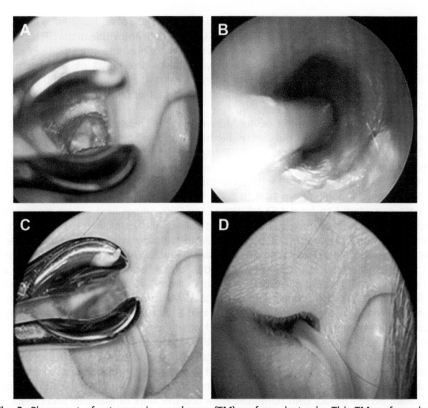

Fig. 3. Placement of a tympanic membrane (TM) surface electrode. This TM surface electrode consists of a soft, hydrogel tip encasing a silver wire threaded through a soft polyethylene tube (TM-ECochGtrode, Bio-logic Systems Corporation/Natus Medical, Mundelein, IL). This electrode is positioned gently onto the central portion of the lateral surface of the TM under microscopic visualization. We use a small nasal or Lempert speculum to avoid dislodging the electrode, as would be the case if a standard ear speculum were used. The electrode is then secured in the canal using the compressible foam tip of the insert transducer used to deliver the auditory stimuli to elicit the response.

disadvantage. This is the preferred recording method in the clinic and operating room at our institution. Recording from the external auditory meatus skin (EAM) can be accomplished with an expanding leaf-type surface electrode or a foam insert earphone covered with gold foil. Although these electrodes are simple to place, the response amplitudes are considerably degraded and the noise levels are higher compared with TM electrodes.

Electrocochleographic Abnormalities in Patients with MD

ECoG is often used in the clinical investigation of hydropic conditions of the cochlea, such as MD, but its diagnostic utility and interpretation remain topics of controversy. The main clinical advantage of ECoG may be the provision of ear-specific information. The characteristic feature of MD is increased SP amplitude relative to AP amplitude.[44,45] It is believed that the presence of hydrops increases the amplitude of the SP by affecting the elasticity and resting position of the basilar membrane, biasing it toward the scala tympani.[46] In addition, as hearing loss progresses, patients with

MD may also have a reduction in AP amplitude owing to loss of auditory nerve fibers.[47] The SP/AP amplitude ratio is used instead of the absolute amplitude of the SP to avoid the effects of interpatient variability and the variability of absolute amplitudes inherent to different measurement techniques. Endolymphatic hydrops is associated with relatively larger SP/AP values. Most investigators have used a value of 0.3 to 0.5 as the upper limit of normal for SP/AP, and have found that approximately two-thirds of MD ears have abnormal ECoG results.[48]

The reported sensitivity of ECoG for MD varies in the literature, in part because the significant overlap of values between patients with and without MD makes it difficult to definitively establish a threshold of SP/AP to consider abnormal. In one study, SP/AP ratios measured for subjects with normal hearing were found to range from 0.04 to 0.59.[49] Gibson and colleagues[50] reported transtympanic SP/AP percentage ratios in healthy subjects ranging from 10% to 63%. Coats and colleagues[51] found that 44% of ears considered to have MD fell below the 95% upper limit values for normal ears. To aid in decision making, Margolis and colleagues[47] published a relatively large series (n = 53) of normative ECoG data. Using tympanic membrane surface electrodes, these investigators found mean click-evoked SP/AP ratios to be dependent on stimulus level, ranging from 0.22 at 78-dB normal hearing level (nHL) to 0.29 at 68-dB nHL. The 95th percentiles of SP/AP ranged from 0.40 to 0.49.[47] By use of similar criteria, with 0.35 or less considered a normal SP/AP and 0.5 or larger for a definitely abnormal test, Pou and colleagues[52] found that 57% of patients with clinically diagnosed endolymphatic hydrops were correctly identified. Using transtympanic ECoG, Ge and Shea[53] reported that an enlarged SP/AP (>0.40) was observed in 1504 of 1976 MD ears (76%). They also noted a significant association between the SP/AP and AAO–HNS stage of disease, degree of hearing loss, and duration of disease. The greater the hearing loss and/or duration of MD, the more often the SP/AP was elevated. Based on our own normative data and the work of Margolis and others,[47] we have defined an SP/AP greater than 0.40 as elevated. **Fig. 2** illustrates an electro-cochleographic recording characterized by an elevated SP/AP ratio obtained from a patient with MD.

Various other approaches aimed at increasing the sensitivity and specificity of ECoG for MD have been proposed. Coats noted that the relationship between SP and AP was nonlinear in healthy subjects, and found that the logarithmic normalization of the SP amplitude by the AP better separated ears with MD from ears with other hearing losses.[44,51] With this technique, 68% of patients with MD had abnormal ECoG and only 7% of non-MD ears were incorrectly identified. Others have advocated for the use of tone-burst stimuli. Margolis and colleagues[47] published normative data on the absolute amplitude of the SP from responses to tone-burst stimuli of 1 kHz (95th percentile from −1.35 to −1.78 μV) and 2-kHz (−1.35 to −2.25 μV). Gibson[54] suggested that measurement of the absolute amplitude of the SP from responses to 1-kHz tone-burst stimuli was optimal, and he considered an SP with an amplitude exceeding 3 μV abnormal. Combining a nonlinear normalization of SP/AP with SP amplitude to tone-bursts, 77% of MD ears were identified correctly and 9% of non-MD ears were identified incorrectly.[54] Conlon and Gibson[55] reported 85% sensitivity for MD ears using 1-kHz tone-bursts. At our institution, we regard an SP amplitude associated with tone-burst stimulation greater than 2 μV to be elevated. Other investigators have proposed that the sensitivity of ECoG may be improved by analyzing the AP latency difference between responses to condensation and rarefaction clicks. In healthy subjects, rarefaction polarity signals produce AP latency values that are slightly shorter than those elicited by condensation polarity signals (mean 0.15–0.27 ms).[47] The AP latency difference has been observed to be significantly larger in MD (95th percentile 0.38 to 0.74 ms) but not in other cochlear disorders.[47,56] At our institution, we consider a significant AP latency difference to be greater than 0.38 ms. Based on observations of a widening of the SP-AP duration in patients with MD, Devaiah and others, working under the guidance of Ferraro,[57] have proposed that the measurement of the area under the SP-AP complex may improve diagnostic sensitivity of ECoG for MD. Further prospective studies will be necessary to determine the measurement(s) that is most sensitive for MD.

It is also important to note that elevation of SP/AP is not specific to MD. Similar ECoG abnormalities have been reported in patients with perilymph fistulae.[58] More recently, Arts and colleagues[59] reported SP/AP elevation (>0.4) in 14 of 15 ears with computed tomographic evidence of superior semicircular canal dehiscence (SSCD), and the SP/AP normalized after canal occlusion. Thus, some patients with an elevated SP/AP and a presentation atypical for MD may actually have SSCD, and it is prudent to exclude this diagnosis before proceeding with MD treatments.

DEHYDRATION TESTING

Although dehydration testing for MD is no longer routinely performed at our institution, there has been renewed interest abroad in examining the effects of acute pharmacologic dehydration on electrocochleography and VEMP measures. Given the apparently successful results of sodium restriction and diuretic therapy in MD, it seems logical that dehydration of the diseased cochlea and labyrinth might reduce endolymphatic volume and hydrops, thus improving peripheral auditory and vestibular function.[60,61]

Armed with an osmotic diuretic known to reduce cerebrospinal fluid and intraocular pressure, Klockhoff and Lindblom[62,63] developed the glycerol dehydration test in 1966. After a baseline audiogram, 3 oz of 95% glycerol mixed with an equal amount of water or juice are served chilled. Repeat audiometric testing is performed if possible at 1 or 2 hours postingestion, and always 3 hours postingestion. The dehydration test has also been attempted with other diuretics, including furosemide, urea, and isosorbide, and through the intravenous route. The test is considered positive if (1) there is a 10-dB or more improvement in pure tone thresholds at 2 or more frequencies (250 to 2000 Hz), or (2) there is a 12% or greater improvement in speech discrimination score. Obviously, hearing loss must be present to have a positive test. The glycerol test is positive in 45% to 60% of patients with a diagnosis of MD, and false positives are rare.[64–66] With furosemide loading, the positive ratio is 55% to 75% of patients with MD.[67–70] The likelihood of a patient having a positive test may depend on the phase of the disease and its fluctuating nature. Tests are more likely to be negative very early (when the membranous labyrinth is normal) and very late in the disease (when the membranous changes are irreversible), although the stage of disease is not predictable purely from dehydration testing.[71]

Critics of dehydration testing note that the tests can be unpleasant, possibly dangerous, insensitive, impractical, and subject to significant placebo effects. Side effects may include headache, nausea, dizziness, diarrhea, thirst, emesis, and diuresis. Glycerol toxicity from overdose has been reported.[72] Nevertheless, there is considerable evidence that a real phenomenon, most likely indicative of endolymphatic hydrops, underlies the test. Indeed, that glycerol dehydration results in improved hearing in a subset of patients with endolymphatic hydrops is regarded as strong evidence that overproduction or impaired reabsorption of endolymph is the underlying pathophysiologic mechanism in MD. Dehydration testing has been revisited in an attempt to improve the sensitivity of VEMP and ECoG.[48,73,74] Whether this modification significantly enhances the sensitivity or specificity of the tests, or if choice of therapy would be altered by the results, remains to be determined.

SUMMARY

Although the AAO–HNS has proposed historical and audiometric criteria for the diagnosis and staging of MD, practitioners often need additional clinical data to make difficult diagnostic and treatment decisions. Vestibular tests can be useful adjuncts in identifying the diseased ear(s) in patients with MD whose symptoms and audiogram are nonlateralizing, for monitoring the development of early disease in the contralateral ear, and for excluding pathology in the contralateral labyrinth in patients who are candidates for ablative therapy. Expanding beyond traditional vestibular evaluations, a "Meniere's-like" response to tone-burst VEMP testing has been identified, and holds promise not only for identifying the diseased ear, but also as a clinical indicator of incipient disease in an asymptomatic ear. As a detector of cochlear disease, the technique of ECoG has been refined and better normative data acquired. The use of ECoG in decision making in patients with MD has evolved beyond the standard assessment of the click-evoked SP/AP to include nonlinear normalization of data, assessment of responses to tone-bursts, AP latency differences, and the area under the SP-AP complex. With these developments in VEMP and ECoG testing, there has been a resurgence in the investigational use of dehydration testing. Nevertheless, no currently available test provides sufficient levels of sensitivity and specificity to be routinely useful for the diagnosis of MD. We are hopeful that ongoing prospective trials will facilitate critical evaluation of our approach to diagnosis, monitoring, and assessment of interventions targeted at halting disease progression.

REFERENCES

1. Ménière P. Memoire sur des lesions de l'oreille interne donnant lieu a des symptomes de congestion cerebrale apoplectiforme. Gazette Medicale de Paris 1861; 16:597–601.
2. Rauch SD, Merchant SN, Thedinger BA. Meniere's syndrome and endolymphatic hydrops. Double-blind temporal bone study. Ann Otol Rhinol Laryngol 1989; 98(11):873–83.
3. Minor L, Schessel D, Carey J. Ménière's disease. Curr Opin Neurol 2004;17(1):9.
4. Merchant S, Adams J, Nadol J. Pathophysiology of Meniere's syndrome: are symptoms caused by endolymphatic hydrops? Otol Neurotol 2005;26(1):74.
5. Committee on Hearing and Equilibrium guidelines for the diagnosis and evaluation of therapy in Ménière's disease. American Academy of Otolaryngology-Head and Neck Foundation, Inc. Otolaryngol Head Neck Surg 1995;113(3):181.
6. Thomas K, Harrison MS. Long-term follow up of 610 cases of Ménière's disease. Proc R Soc Med 1971;64(8):853.
7. Green JD, Blum DJ, Harner SG. Longitudinal followup of patients with Menière's disease. Otolaryngol Head Neck Surg 1991;104(6):783.
8. Haye R, Quist-Hanssen S. The natural course of Meniere's disease. Acta Otolaryngol 1976;82(3–4):289.
9. Paparella MM, McDermott JC, de Sousa LC. Meniere's disease and the peak audiogram. Arch Otolaryngol 1982;108(9):555.
10. Stahle J, Friberg U, Svedberg A. Long-term progression of Meniere's disease. Am J Otol 1989;10(3):170–3.

11. Mateijsen DJ, Van Hengel PW, Van Huffelen WM, et al. Pure-tone and speech audiometry in patients with Meniere's disease. Clin Otolaryngol Allied Sci 2001; 26(5):379–87.
12. Stahle J. Advanced Meniere's disease. A study of 356 severely disabled patients. Acta Otolaryngol 1976;81(1–2):113.
13. Muchnik C, Hildesheimer M, Rubinstein M, et al. Low frequency air-bone gap in Menière's disease without middle ear pathology. A preliminary report. Am J Otol 1989; 10(1):1.
14. Hallpike CS, Hood JD. Observations upon the neurological mechanism of the loudness recruitment phenomenon. Acta Otolaryngol 1959;50:472–86.
15. Dimitri PS, Wall C 3rd, Rauch SD. Multivariate vestibular testing: laterality of unilateral Meniere's disease. J Vestib Res 2001;11(6):405–12.
16. Dimitri PS, Wall C 3rd, Rauch SD. Multivariate vestibular testing: thresholds for bilateral Meniere's disease and aminoglycoside ototoxicity. J Vestib Res 2001; 11(6):391–404.
17. Enander A, Stahle J. Hearing loss and caloric response in Meniere's disease. A comparative study. Acta Otolaryngol 1969;67(1):57–68.
18. Black FO, Kitch R. A review of vestibular test results in Meniere's disease. Otolaryngol Clin North Am 1980;13(4):631–42.
19. Park HJ, Migliaccio AA, Della Santina CC, et al. Search-coil head-thrust and caloric tests in Meniere's disease. Acta Otolaryngol 2005;125(8):852–7.
20. Katsarkas A. Hearing loss and vestibular dysfunction in Meniere's disease. Acta Otolaryngol 1996;116(2):185–8.
21. Maire R, van Melle G. Vestibulo-ocular reflex characteristics in patients with unilateral Meniere's disease. Otol Neurotol 2008;29(5):693–8.
22. Proctor LR. Results of serial vestibular testing in unilateral Meniere's disease. Am J Otol 2000;21(4):552–8.
23. Rizvi SS. Investigations into the cause of canal paresis in Meniere's disease. Laryngoscope 1986;96(11):1258–71.
24. Beck C, Schmidt CL. 10 years of experience with intratympanally applied streptomycin (gentamycin) in the therapy of Morbus Meniere. Arch Otorhinolaryngol 1978;221(2):149–52.
25. Minor LB. Intratympanic gentamicin for control of vertigo in Meniere's disease: vestibular signs that specify completion of therapy. Am J Otol 1999;20(2):209–19.
26. Palomar-Asenjo V, Boleas-Aguirre MS, Sanchez-Ferrandiz N, et al. Caloric and rotatory chair test results in patients with Meniere's disease. Otol Neurotol 2006;27(7):945–50.
27. Mateijsen DJ, Hengel PW, Kingma H, et al. Vertigo and electronystagmography in uni- and bilateral Meniere's disease. ORL J Otorhinolaryngol Relat Spec 2001; 63(6):341–8.
28. Schuknecht HF. Meniere's disease: a correlation of symptomatology and pathology. Laryngoscope 1963;73:651.
29. Guyot JP, Psillas G. Test-retest reliability of vestibular autorotation testing in healthy subjects. Otolaryngol Head Neck Surg 1997;117(6):704–7.
30. Soto A, Labella T, Santos S, et al. The usefulness of computerized dynamic posturography for the study of equilibrium in patients with Meniere's disease: correlation with clinical and audiologic data. Hear Res 2004;196(1–2):26–32.
31. Colebatch JG, Halmagyi GM, Skuse NF. Myogenic potentials generated by a click-evoked vestibulocollic reflex. J Neurol Neurosurg Psychiatry 1994;57(2):190–7.
32. Zhou G, Cox LC. Vestibular evoked myogenic potentials: history and overview. Am J Audiol 2004;13(2):135–43.

33. Kushiro K, Zakir M, Ogawa Y, et al. Saccular and utricular inputs to sternocleido-mastoid motoneurons of decerebrate cats. Exp Brain Res 1999;126(3):410–6.
34. Schuknecht HF. Endolymphatic hydrops: can it be controlled? Ann Otol Rhinol Laryngol 1986;95(1 Pt 1):36–9.
35. Rauch S, Zhou G, Kujawa S, et al. Vestibular evoked myogenic potentials show altered tuning in patients with Ménière's disease. Otol Neurotol 2004;25(3):333.
36. Cheng PW, Huang TW, Young YH. The influence of clicks versus short tone bursts on the vestibular evoked myogenic potentials. Ear Hear 2003;24(3):195–7.
37. de Waele C, Huy PT, Diard JP, et al. Saccular dysfunction in Meniere's disease. Am J Otol 1999;20(2):223–32.
38. Murofushi T, Shimizu K, Takegoshi H, et al. Diagnostic value of prolonged laten-cies in the vestibular evoked myogenic potential. Arch Otolaryngol Head Neck Surg 2001;127(9):1069–72.
39. Janky KL, Shepard N. Vestibular evoked myogenic potential (VEMP) testing: normative threshold response curves and effects of age. J Am Acad Audiol 2009;20(8):514–22.
40. Lin M, Timmer FCA, Oriel B, et al. Vestibular evoked myogenic potentials (VEMP) can detect asymptomatic saccular hydrops. Laryngoscope 2006;116(6):987.
41. Rauch SD, Silveira MB, Zhou G, et al. Vestibular evoked myogenic potentials versus vestibular test battery in patients with Meniere's disease. Otol Neurotol 2004;25(6):981–6.
42. Dallos P, Wang CY. Bioelectric correlates of kanamycin intoxication. Audiology 1974;13(4):277.
43. Durrant JD, Wang J, Ding DL, et al. Are inner or outer hair cells the source of summating potentials recorded from the round window? J Acoust Soc Am 1998;104(1):370.
44. Coats AC. The summating potential and Meniere's disease. I. Summating poten-tial amplitude in Meniere and non-Meniere ears. Arch Otolaryngol 1981;107(4):199–208.
45. Dauman R, Aran JM, Charlet de Sauvage R, et al. Clinical significance of the summating potential in Meniere's disease. Am J Otol 1988;9(1):31–8.
46. Durrant JD, Dallos P. Modification of DIF summating potential components by stimulus biasing. J Acoust Soc Am 1974;56(2):562–70.
47. Margolis RH, Rieks D, Fournier EM, et al. Tympanic electrocochleography for diagnosis of Meniere's disease. Arch Otolaryngol Head Neck Surg 1995;121(1):44–55.
48. Aso S, Watanabe Y, Mizukoshi K. A clinical study of electrocochleography in Meniere's disease. Acta Otolaryngol 1991;111(1):44–52.
49. Chatrian GE, Wirch AL, Edwards KH, et al. Cochlear summating potential to broadband clicks detected from the human external auditory meatus. A study of subjects with normal hearing for age. Ear Hear 1985;6(3):130–8.
50. Gibson WP, Prasher DK, Kilkenny GP. Diagnostic significance of transtympanic electrocochleography in Meniere's disease. Ann Otol Rhinol Laryngol 1983;92(2 Pt 1):155–9.
51. Coats AC, Jenkins HA, Monroe B. Auditory evoked potentials—the cochlear summating potential in detection of endolymphatic hydrops. Am J Otol 1984;5(6):443–6.
52. Pou AM, Hirsch BE, Durrant JD, et al. The efficacy of tympanic electrocochleog-raphy in the diagnosis of endolymphatic hydrops. Am J Otol 1996;17(4):607–11.
53. Ge X, Shea JJ Jr. Transtympanic electrocochleography: a 10-year experience. Otol Neurotol 2002;23(5):799–805.

54. Gibson WP. The use of electrocochleography in the diagnosis of Meniere's disease. Acta Otolaryngol Suppl 1991;485:46–52.
55. Conlon BJ, Gibson WP. Electrocochleography in the diagnosis of Meniere's disease. Acta Otolaryngol 2000;120(4):480.
56. Levine SC, Margolis RH, Fournier EM, et al. Tympanic electrocochleography for evaluation of endolymphatic hydrops. Laryngoscope 1992;102(6):614.
57. Devaiah AK, Dawson KL, Ferraro JA, et al. Utility of area curve ratio electrocochleography in early Meniere disease. Arch Otolaryngol Head Neck Surg 2003; 129(5):547–51.
58. Arenberg IK, Ackley RS, Ferraro J, et al. ECoG results in perilymphatic fistula: clinical and experimental studies. Otolaryngol Head Neck Surg 1988;99(5):435.
59. Arts HA, Adams M, Telian S, et al. Reversible electrocochleographic abnormalities in superior canal dehiscence. Otol Neurotol 2009;30(1):79.
60. Boles R, Rice DH, Hybels R, et al. Conservative management of Meniere's disease: Furstenberg regimen revisited. Ann Otol Rhinol Laryngol 1975;84(4 Pt 1):513–7.
61. Klockhoff I, Lindblom U, Stahle J. Diuretic treatment of Meniere disease. Long-term results with chlorthalidone. Arch Otolaryngol 1974;100(4):262–5.
62. Klockhoff I, Lindblom U. Endolymphatic hydrops revealed by glycerol test. Preliminary report. Acta Otolaryngol 1966;61(5):459–62.
63. Klockhoff I, Lindblom U. Glycerol test in Meniere's disease. Acta Otolaryngol 1966;(Suppl 224):449+.
64. Snyder JM. Extensive use of a diagnostic test for Meniere disease. Arch Otolaryngol 1974;100(5):360–5.
65. Akioka K, Fujita N, Kitaoku Y. A clinical study of the diagnosis of the endolymphatic hydrops aspect of Meniere's disease. In: Kitahara M, editor. Meniere's Disease. Tokyo: Springer-Verlag; 1990. p. 125–32.
66. Stahle J, Klockhoff I. Diagnostic procedures, differential diagnosis, and general conclusions. In: Pfaltz C, editor. Controversial aspects of Meniere disease. New York: Thieme, Inc; 1986. p. 71–86.
67. Mori N, Asai A, Suizu Y, et al. Comparison between electrocochleography and glycerol test in the diagnosis of Meniere's disease. Scand Audiol 1985;14(4):209–13.
68. Aso S, Kimura H, Takeda S, et al. The intravenously administered glycerol test. Acta Otolaryngol Suppl 1993;504:51–4.
69. Futaki T, Kitahara M, Morimoto M. A comparison of the furosemide and glycerol tests for Meniere's disease. With special reference to the bilateral lesion. Acta Otolaryngol 1977;83(3–4):272–8.
70. Tsunoda R, Fukaya T, Komatsuzaki A. The furosemide test and vestibular status in Meniere's disease. Acta Otolaryngol 1998;118(2):157–60.
71. Karjalainen S, Krj J, Nuutinen J. The limited value of the glycerol test in Menière's disease. J Laryngol Otol 1984;98(3):259.
72. Andresen H, Bingel U, Streichert T, et al. Severe glycerol intoxication after Menière's disease diagnostic—case report and overview of kinetic data. Clin Toxicol 2009;47(4):312.
73. Seo T, Node M, Yukimasa A, et al. Furosemide loading vestibular evoked myogenic potential for unilateral Meniere's disease. Otol Neurotol 2003; 24(2):283–8.
74. Shojaku H, Takemori S, Kobayashi K, et al. Clinical usefulness of glycerol vestibular-evoked myogenic potentials: preliminary report. Acta Otolaryngol Suppl 2001;545:65–8.

Clinical Hints and Precipitating Factors in Patients Suffering from Meniere's Disease

Steven D. Rauch, MD

KEYWORDS

• Meniere's disease • Vertigo • Migraine

Meniere's disease is one of the most fascinating and most vexing of all clinical conditions encountered by the otolaryngologist. Despite having captivated the interest of clinicians and researchers for a century and a half and thousands of papers having been written about it, the causes, pathophysiology, and treatments of Meniere's disease are not completely understood. Nonetheless, there is merit in occasionally taking inventory of the many findings and developments in inner ear research to update our thinking about this disorder of hearing and balance.

TOWARD A MODERN DEFINITION OF MENIERE'S DISEASE

The nomenclature of Meniere's "disease" versus Meniere's "syndrome" in the otolaryngology literature is confusing enough and is not revisited here. Meniere's disease is a "phenotype"; that is, it is a clinical presentation of unstable hearing and balance that may arise from many different insults to the inner ear. There is compelling evidence that it can arise from genetic factors, inflammatory and immunologic dysfunction, infection, trauma, and vasculopathy. Disturbances of barometric pressure, osmotic pressure, hydrostatic pressure, and perfusion pressure have all been incriminated at one time or another as factors in Meniere's disease. A normal ear has a host of homeostatic systems. These systems regulate the production, maintenance, and recycling of endolymph and perilymph. They regulate efferent and afferent nerve signaling, efferent and afferent blood flow, intercellular signaling, ion cycling, mitochondrial energy metabolism, and other processes. Under normal circumstances, these homeostatic systems are so robust that inner ear functions of hearing and balance are impervious to changes in the rest of the body or the external environment. In Meniere's disease one or more of these systems is dysfunctional. As a consequence of impaired homeostasis, hearing and balance functions become vulnerable to myriad internal and

Otology and Laryngology, Harvard Medical School, Massachusetts Eye and Ear Infirmary, 243 Charles Street, Boston, MA 02114, USA
E-mail address: steven_rauch@meei.harvard.edu

Otolaryngol Clin N Am 43 (2010) 1011–1017
doi:10.1016/j.otc.2010.05.003
0030-6665/10/$ – see front matter © 2010 Elsevier Inc. All rights reserved.

external factors, such as stress, sleep deprivation, dietary indiscretion, hormonal change, allergies, and barometric pressure change. Operationally speaking, a Meniere's ear is a fragile ear. In fact, Meniere's disease can and should be redefined as a degenerating inner ear that has impairment of one of more homeostatic systems resulting in instability of hearing and balance function (**Fig. 1**).

APPLICATION OF THE MODERN DEFINITION OF MENIERE'S DISEASE—DIAGNOSIS

There are 2 reasons to assign a patient's condition a specific diagnosis: (1) to guide treatment and (2) to prognosticate. The American Academy of Otolaryngology–Head and Neck Surgery (AAO-HNS) Hearing and Equilibrium Subcommittee has published guidelines for the classification and reporting of Meniere's disease treatment outcomes.[1] These guidelines specify character, frequency, and duration of vertigo attacks necessary to achieve a diagnosis of Meniere's disease. These guidelines have been updated periodically, with the last update in 1995. Although adoption of standardized diagnostic and reporting criteria are essential in research studies, one can afford to be somewhat less dogmatic in routine clinical practice. The 2 critical features of the Meniere's phenotype that enable diagnosis are (1) instability and (2) involvement of both hearing and balance. Patients with isolated hearing instability or isolated vestibular symptoms do not meet Meniere's diagnostic criteria. The old nomenclature of "cochlear Meniere's" and "vestibular Meniere's" was abandoned with the 1985 update of AAO-HNS criteria because there is insufficient evidence that these entities share essential pathophysiology with Meniere's disease and because many such patients never meet Meniere's criteria for involvement of auditory and vestibular systems.

Patients with Meniere's disease exhibit huge variability in symptoms, within and between patients. Symptoms may occur in clusters or sporadically. Patients may have a great deal of hearing fluctuation or rapid loss but relatively infrequent vertigo ("auditory dominant" pattern), frequent and severe vertigo attacks but only mild hearing loss or infrequent fluctuations ("vestibular dominant" pattern), or auditory and vestibular symptoms that occur together or with relatively equal frequency and severity ("mixed" pattern). Although these patterns seem evident clinically, they have never been characterized epidemiologically. It is not known if there are 3 distinct pattern

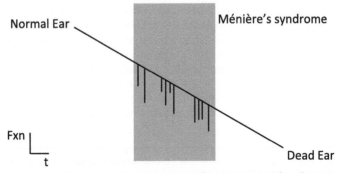

Meniere's = Unstable Inner Ear

Normal Ear

Ménière's syndrome

Fxn

t

Dead Ear

Fig. 1. The diagnosis of Meniere's disease is assigned to patients with a degenerating inner ear who have developed instability of hearing and balance function. The ear may have been degenerating for months or years before achieving the diagnosis and may continue to degenerate after the hearing and balance functions have "burnt out" and episodic symptoms ceased. Fxn, inner ear function; t, time.

classes or a continuum. Nor is it known if patients remain "true to class" over time or if they transition from one class to another. If there are class transitions, it is not known if all patients pass through the classes in the same order. It is also not known if these different pattern classes indicate specific underlying pathophysiologic mechanisms or causes. The current best practice is to consider patients with combined auditory and vestibular instability to be patients with Meniere's disease and treat them accordingly.

APPLICATION OF THE MODERN DEFINITION OF MENIERE'S DISEASE—TREATMENT

Traditionally, Meniere's disease has been treated with dietary restriction of sodium, caffeine, and alcohol; with diuretics; and with invasive procedures. Since Hallpike and Cairns[2] and Yamakawa[3] first reported endolymphatic hydrops in postmortem examination of temporal bones of patients with Meniere's disease, there was a presumption that endolymphatic hydrops caused the fluctuating progressive hearing loss and vertigo attacks of Meniere's disease. Recommendation to restrict sodium intake was originally conceived as a way of reducing "fluid retention" in the inner ear. Although this notion might seem simplistic and improbable, the fact is that many patients with Meniere's disease are sensitive to sodium intake and do better on a restricted diet. Likewise, diuretics were first proposed to reduce endolymph volume. It is impossible to imagine that someone on a diuretic is urinating endolymph, but many patients with Meniere's disease seem to improve on diuretic therapy.[4–6] The modern definition of Meniere's disease offers an explanation. A normal ear has homeostatic mechanisms that keep the fluid and electrolyte status of the inner ear tightly controlled and stable. A Meniere's ear has lost this regulatory control. Diet and diuretic therapy place the responsibility for regulatory control in the patient's hands and are means of pampering the fragile ear. A fragile ear may be intolerant of variations in sodium levels. If so, it is likely that a low sodium level is not actually the important feature of treatment. A constant sodium level is the critical feature. By evening out sodium intake across the day, patients reduce the risk of spikes that trigger symptoms. Although a very low sodium diet will achieve even distribution through the day, an even distribution can also be maintained on a "no added salt" (NAS) diet of 2000 to 3000 mg sodium per day. A target of 500 to 1000 mg of sodium per meal is relatively easy to achieve. Patient compliance is much better on the NAS diet than on a more severe restriction. There is an additional benefit of the more modest sodium restriction. If a patient is used to an extremely low sodium diet, a single handful of potato chips may double their day's sodium intake, a spike that could easily trigger an attack. Alternatively, if the patient is equilibrated on the NAS diet of 1000 mg/meal, that same handful of chips may be only a 25% to 30% increase rather than 100% increase in daily sodium. The spike is relatively smaller and thus less likely to trigger symptoms.

Perspiring and subsequent fluid replacement is another potential source of inner ear stress that could trigger Meniere's attacks. Maintenance of a stable fluid and electrolyte status is a primary objective in this updated approach to Meniere's management. Therefore, in our clinic we stress that when patients with Meniere's disease perspire, it is important that they actively replace their fluid loss with a sports drink or other electrolyte solution. The patients are perspiring saltwater, which must be replaced with something comparable. Patients are advised to sip the replacement solution frequently as they perspire, rather than dehydrating for an hour and then replacing with a single large bolus of fluid. For a 75-kg man perspiring freely, replacement rate is approximately 1 L/h. Sodium intake during fluid replacement while perspiring is not counted in the day's total because it is canceled out by the loss through perspiration.

Caffeine and alcohol cause large fluid shifts through physiologic fluid compartments. Limiting their use to no more than a single "dose" per day is another way to keep the inner ear stable and avoid triggering an attack. Diuretics affect ion pumps and ionic gradients in the ear as well as in the kidney. It is likely that diuretic therapy in Meniere's disease works via its influence on inner fluid and electrolyte processing and not by dehydrating the inner ear through inducing urination of endolymph. The guiding principle in all the conservative medical treatments with dietary restrictions, fluid replacement, and diuretics is to reduce stress on the inner ear's fluid and electrolyte status so that it can retain a sufficient degree of stability.

Many of the other triggers for Meniere's attacks, such as stress, hormonal change, barometric pressure change, sleep deprivation, and allergy attacks, can all be seen as challenges to the homeostasis of the fragile Meniere's ear. Thus, patients with Meniere's disease seem to do best if they have a regular daily routine, with meals at the same time each day, plenty of sleep, and some regular exercise. Patients with Meniere's disease also do better if they have good general health and if they work with their primary care physician and other doctors to manage any other health issues. Common general health issues whose management often benefits the patient with Meniere's disease include sleep disorders, allergies, thyroid dysfunction, diabetes, and perimenstrual or peripmenopausal hormonal fluctuations.

TREATMENT EFFECTIVENESS

Meniere's disease is a failure of homeostasis in a degenerating inner ear resulting in instability of hearing and balance function. This instability may arise from a host of different causes. By the time patients meet diagnostic criteria for Meniere's disease, the ear is already significantly damaged. If faltering homeostasis could be detected while the causative process was still in evidence, perhaps it could be treated specifically. However, this is not possible at the present time. We are therefore left with "palliative" therapy.

Treatments for Meniere's disease are very effective for management of vertigo. Diet and lifestyle measures achieve vertigo control in up to two-thirds of patients. Diuretic therapy helps achieve vertigo control in approximately two-thirds of those who fail the diet and lifestyle treatments. Only a small group of patients, 5% to 10% of the total, who continue to have intractable vertigo require invasive therapy. Invasive treatment options, including Meniett pump, endolymphatic sac surgery, intratympanic steroids or intratympanic gentamicin injections, vestibular neurectomy, and labyrinthectomy, achieve vertigo control in 99% of this last group of intractable patients. Thus, vertigo is ultimately controlled in more than 99% of patients with Meniere's disease.

Unfortunately, treatments for Meniere's disease appear to offer little predictable benefit for auditory symptoms of aural fullness, tinnitus, and fluctuating progressive sensorineural hearing loss.[7] The intrusiveness of the aural fullness and tinnitus can be highly variable. Hearing loss may progress stepwise or continuously and it may drop either slowly or rapidly. But regardless of treatment, the vast majority of patients with Meniere's disease gradually lose hearing in the affected ear.

MIGRAINE AND MENIERE'S DISEASE

Over the last 25 years, there has been an increasing awareness and acceptance of migraine as a cause of dizziness, imbalance, and vertigo. Traditionally, migraine has been considered as a headache disorder, with adjunctive symptoms, including scintillating scotomata and other ocular manifestations, photophobia and/or phonophobia, nausea and vomiting, and allodynia (tactile hypersensitivity or pain produced by nonnoxious stimuli on the skin). This conception dominates the migraine literature and the education of neurologists. However, there is clinical and basic science evidence that migraine is actually a global disturbance of sensory perception arising from abnormal processing of neurotransmitters and resulting in a broad spectrum of sensory distortions and intensifications. Large epidemiologic studies have shown that 25% to 35% of migraineurs experience episodes of dizziness or vertigo, many of which are indistinguishable from Meniere's attacks.[8] Animal studies[9,10] have shown trigeminovascular control of cochlear blood flow, and clinical reports[11,12] suggest that as many as 25% of migraineurs may experience fluctuating or progressive sensorineural hearing loss. It is virtually certain that a significant subset of "classic" Meniere's disease cases is migrainous. Migraine should therefore be added to the list of putative causes of Meniere's disease.

The overall prevalence of migraine in the general population is 13%,[13] and 25% of those patients (3.25% of the general population) experience dizziness or vertigo along with other migraine symptoms. Because the prevalence of Meniere's disease in the general population has been estimated at only 0.2% to 0.5%,[14] a patient presenting with episodic vertigo is up to 15 times more likely to have migraine-associated vertigo than Meniere's disease. How many practicing otolaryngologists are currently diagnosing migraine 15 times more often than Meniere's disease? On a purely statistical basis, one would predict that 13% of patients with Meniere's disease would also be migraineurs. In fact, the comorbidity of Meniere's disease and migraine is much higher. The prevalence of migraine in patients with Meniere's disease is 56%, and in patients with bilateral Meniere's disease, it is 85%.[15]

If migraine-associated vertigo is so much more common than Meniere's disease and if the symptoms overlap so heavily, how does one differentiate them? When does a patient have simple Meniere's disease? When do they have migraine-associated vertigo? When do they have migrainous Meniere's disease and when is migraine present as an unrelated health issue? Meniere's disease is an inner ear disorder. Migraine is a neurologic disorder with possible inner ear manifestations. There is no doubt that many patients diagnosed with "atypical Meniere's" are actually migraineurs. Patients with Meniere's disease always have associated hearing loss in one ear; migraineurs may not. Patients with simple Meniere's disease do not have migraine headaches temporally associated with their vertigo attacks. They do not have scintillating scotomata, photophobia, or phonophobia. They rarely complain of the cognitive dysfunction ("brain fog") that is prevalent in migraineurs. Patients with Meniere's disease typically only feel nauseous during a vertigo attack. In contrast, migraineurs are plagued by many smoldering sensory symptoms. Even when they are not in the throes of an acute vertigo attack, they may have "rocking boat" disequilibrium, nausea, motion intolerance, and brain fog. They often admit to photophobia and/or phonophobia that accompany their acute vertigo attacks. They often have vertigo attacks in close temporal association with headache or ocular migraine. Migraine has a significant genetic component, and many migraineurs have other affected family members. Migraineurs are sensitive to diet, barometric pressure change, stress, lack of sleep, hunger or dehydration, and hormonal fluctuation.

Early in the assessment and management of a patient with possible Meniere's disease, differentiating Meniere's disease from migraine may not be all that important. The lifestyle recommendations of regular meals, sleep, and exercise and the general medical management of any other outstanding health issues benefit both conditions. However, the treatments of migraine and Meniere's disease diverge at this point. Both conditions respond to dietary modification, but a migraine diet is drastically different from a Meniere's diet restricted in salt, caffeine, and alcohol. Because invasive therapies for Meniere's disease, such as endolymphatic sac surgery and intratympanic gentamicin injections, are irreversible, it is most critical to differentiate migraine from Meniere's disease when conservative and medical measures of treatment have failed and one is considering one of these invasive options. If migraine is at all a possibility, at this point in the management, it is prudent to offer patients a trial of aggressive migraine management. A 1- to 2-month trial of strict migraine diet and lifestyle is undertaken first. If this trial fails to gain adequate symptom control, patients are continued on the diet and a migraine suppressant medication is added. Migraineurs tend to be extremely susceptible to medication side effects, so suppressants are best started at a subtherapeutic dose and increased in small increments every 2 weeks. It typically takes about 6 to 8 weeks to reach a reasonable therapeutic dose and determine if the medication is helping. Further dose adjustment may be needed, but usually there is some indication within 2 months that the treatment is on the right track. If there is no indication of symptom response to migraine therapy, then invasive treatment for Meniere's disease can be undertaken with confidence.

SUMMARY

The modern conception of Meniere's disease is that of unstable hearing and balance arising from a failure of inner ear homeostasis in a damaged or degenerating inner ear. By the time the diagnosis is achieved, the actual causative process may no longer be in evidence, so treatments are palliative, seeking to pamper the fragile inner ear to minimize vestibular symptoms or disable the symptomatic ear that does not respond to pampering. Conservative treatments include lifestyle and dietary adjustments, diuretics, and supplemental use of vestibular suppressants. Invasive or destructive procedures are indicated only in the 5% to 10% of patients with Meniere's disease who fail conservative and medical measures. Overall, vertigo control is achieved in more than 99% of patients with Meniere's disease. Unfortunately, auditory symptoms of progressive hearing loss, aural fullness, and tinnitus tend to be minimally responsive to treatment. Eventual involvement of the second ear is seen in 25% to 35% of patients with Meniere's disease. The treatment algorithm is the same for the second ear. However, because there is no stable contralateral inner ear, patients with bilateral Meniere's disease tend to have worse symptoms before treatment and more residual imbalance after treatment. They also eventually require some sort of hearing hardware, either hearing aids or cochlear implants.

REFERENCES

1. Committee on Hearing and Equilibrium guidelines for the diagnosis and evaluation of therapy in Meniere's disease. American Academy of Otolaryngology-Head and Neck Foundation, Inc. Otolaryngol Head Neck Surg 1995;113:181–5.
2. Hallpike CS, Cairns H. Observations on the pathology Meniere's syndrome. J Laryngol Otol 1938;53:625–55.
3. Yamakawa K. Über die pathologische Veränderung bei einem Meniere-Kranken. J Otorhinolaryngol Soc Jpn 1938;44:2310–2 [in German].
4. Klockoff I, Lindblom U. Meniere's disease and hydrochlorothiazide (Dichlotride) – a critical analysis of symptoms and therapeutic effects. Acta Otolaryngol 1967; 63:347–65.
5. Van Deelen GW, Huizing EH. Use of a diuretic (Dyazide) in the treatment of Meniere's disease. A double-blind cross-over placebo-controlled study. ORL J Otorhinolaryngol Relat Spec 1986;48:287–92.

6. Santos PM, Hall RA, Snyder JM, et al. Diuretic and diet effect on Meniere's disease evaluated by the 1985 Committee on Hearing and Equilibrium guidelines. Otolaryngol Head Neck Surg 1993;109:680–9.
7. Kinney S, Sandridge S, Newman C. Long-term effects of Meniere's disease on hearing and quality of life. Am J Otol 1997;18:67–73.
8. Kayan A, Hood JD. Neuro-otological manifestations of migraine. Brain 1984; 107(Pt 4):1123–42.
9. Vass Z, Shore SE, Nuttall AL, et al. Trigeminal ganglion innervation of the cochlea – a retrograde transport study. Neuroscience 1997;79:605–15.
10. Vass Z, Shore SE, Nuttall AL, et al. Direct evidence of trigeminal innervation of the cochlear blood vessels. Neuroscience 1998;84:559–67.
11. Lee H, Ishiyama A, Baloh RW. Can migraine damage the inner ear? Arch Neurol 2000;57:1631–4.
12. Virre ES, Baloh RW. Migraine as a cause of sudden hearing loss. Headache 1996; 36:24–8.
13. Lipton RB, Stewart WF, Diamond S, et al. Prevalence and burden of migraine in the United States: data from the American Migraine Study II. Headache 2001; 41:646–57.
14. Stahle J, Stahle C, Arenberg IK. Incidence of Meniere's disease. Arch Otolaryngol 1978;104:99–102.
15. Wladislavosky-Waserman P, Facer G, Mokri B, et al. Meniere's disease: a 30-year epidemiologic and clinical study in Rochester, MN 1951–1980. Laryngoscope 1984;94:1098–102.

Hypothetical Mechanism for Vertigo in Meniere's Disease

William P.R. Gibson, MD, FRCS, FRACS[a,b,*]

KEYWORDS

- Meniere's disease • Endolymph • Hydrops
- Vertigo • Dizziness • Vestibular system

Vertigo is the major symptom of Meniere's disease during the early stages of the disorder. The vertigo can be very unpleasant and disabling and can occur with little warning. Characteristically there is a sensation of movement, usually a feeling of rotation, associated with nausea and vomiting. Each attack occurs for at least 10 minutes and may last for several hours. Each attack is separated from the next by at least one day. The attacks of vertigo tend to occur in clusters over a period of several weeks followed by variable periods of remission. Sometimes the periods of remission may last for several years, or the disorder may completely resolve.

Understanding the pathophysiological mechanism that causes the attacks of vertigo could provide the key to understanding the etiology of Meniere's disease.

Before Prosper Ménière's[1] classic description of the disease, it was thought the vertigo attacks were caused by cerebral apoplexy or a type of epilepsy. Ménière correctly attributed the attacks to a disorder of the inner ear, but his original paper was met with scorn and skepticism. Ménière suggested the mechanism could be similar to migraine, and for a while the popular theory was that vasospasm within the inner ear caused the attacks. Different therapies were based on this hypothesis, including cervical sympathectomy and vasodilator medications such as nicotinic acid.[2]

In 1938, Hallpike and Cairns[3] in London and Kyoshiro Yamakawa[4] in Japan both independently published temporal bone histologic studies that showed the presence of endolymphatic hydrops. Endolymphatic hydrops is a term to describe increased volume of endolymph within the membranous inner ear. It also was commonly supposed that there was an increased pressure of endolymph causing the attacks.

[a] Department of Surgery/Otolaryngology, The University of Sydney, New South Wales 2006, Australia
[b] The Royal prince Alfred Hospital, Sydney The Children's Hospital, Westmead, New South Wales, Australia
* Suite 7, 155 Missenden Road, Newtown 2042, Australia.
E-mail address: wpr_gibson@bigpond.com

Otolaryngol Clin N Am 43 (2010) 1019–1027
doi:10.1016/j.otc.2010.05.013
0030-6665/10/$ – see front matter Crown Copyright © 2010 Published by Elsevier Inc. All rights reserved.

In 1964, Schuknecht[5] proposed the rupture theory, based on his histologic studies, where he identified areas of Reissner membrane that showed evidence of healing after ruptures. He suggested that these might have occurred because of increased endolymph volume and that the ruptures in Reissner membrane led to mixing of potassium-rich endolymph with perilymph. The afferent vestibular nerves were paralyzed by the high potassium until the ionic pumps within the inner ear restored the electrolyte levels and the rupture healed.

The rupture theory remained the most plausible explanation for several decades. The theory led to the concept that it was blockage of flow along the endolymphatic duct that led to endolymphatic hydrops.[6] Endolymphatic sac surgery was believed to unblock the duct and allow the endolymphatic sac to function effectively again, clearing the excess endolymph and restoring normal inner ear function.

As knowledge of the physiology and pathophysiology of the ear has developed over recent years, the original rupture theory hypothesis has seemed increasingly unlikely, and alternative theories have evolved to explain a sudden potassium contamination of the perilymph. For example, leakage of potassium through gaps in the tight junctions and changes in the calcium levels controlling tight junctions in vestibular hair cells have been suggested.[7] But is the vertigo truly a result of potassium leakage, or should an alternative hypothesis be sought? The anatomy and physiology of the inner ear are complex. Great strides in understanding have occurred, however, and this must be considered before formulating any hypothesis (**Fig. 1**).

THE ANATOMY OF THE ENDOLYMPHATIC SAC AND DUCT

The anatomy of the human endolymphatic duct and sac is shown in **Fig. 1**. The duct begins at the ductus reuniens, which joins the cochlear duct and the utricle to form an endolymphatic duct (ED) leading to the endolymphatic sac (ELS). The anatomy has been described by Lo and his colleagues.[8] Often anatomic texts describe a long thin ED ending in a short, pouch-like ELS, but in reality, the system is far different in appearance. The ED is a short single-lumen tube of only 2 mm in length. The ELS is

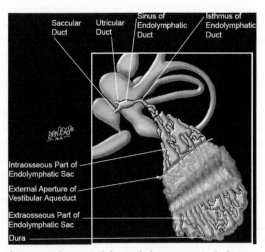

Fig. 1. A diagram of the membranous labyrinth (pars superior). (*From* Lo WM, Daniels DL, Chakeres DW, et al. The endolymphatic sac and duct. AJNR Am J Neuroradiol 1997;18:881–7; with permission. Copyright © 1997 American Society of Neuroradiology.)

much larger and a highly complex structure of interconnecting tubules, cisterns and crypts. The endolymphatic sinus (ES) lies in a groove on the posteromedial surface of the vestibule, with its distal outlet leading to the vestibular aqueduct. The ED narrows at its isthmus at the isthmus of the vestibular aqueduct (VA), where it is oblong in shape with mean diameter of only 0.09 × 0.2 mm. Distal to the isthmus begins the ELS, which flares considerably transversely but thickens only slightly in its sagittal dimension. The ELS has two portions, the intraosseous portion within the VA, and the extraosseous portion. The size of the intraosseous portion varies considerably, from 6 to 15 mm in length and 3 to 15 mm in width. The extraosseous ELS rests on a fovea on the posterior wall of the petrous bone, where the ELS lies between two layers of dura. The extraosseous ELS also varies considerably in size, from 5 to 7 mm in width and 10 to 15 mm in length.

In lower animals and the human fetus, the ELS consists of a single lumen. In people after the age of 1 year, the ELS develops tubules that reach adult complexity by the age of 3 to 4 years. The tubules of the ELS are more complex in the proximal and middle (rugose) portions. The concept of the human ELS as a empty sack is entirely wrong.

The bony (VA) has a smaller diameter in Meniere's ears than the median in normal ears.[9] Basically all Meniere's ears have a small VA, but there are non-Meniere's ears that also have small-diameter VA.

THE PHYSIOLOGY OF THE ENDOLYMPHATIC SAC AND ITS ROLE IN LONGITUDINAL ENDOLYMPH FLOW

The ELS has absorptive and secretory functions as well as phagocytic and immune defence functions.[10] It has been known for many years that debris placed into the cochlear duct passes to the ELS. How the debris reaches the endolymphatic sac has been a matter of conjecture but there must be longitudinal flow of endolymph.

The endolymphatic sac secretes various substances, including aquaporins,[11] glycoproteins,[12] and even endolymph. Glycoprotein is highly hydrophilic, and studies suggest that when longitudinal flow occurs, the glycoprotein is rapidly eaten away by phagocytic activity. It is possible that the glycoprotein is both produced and eaten away to cause longitudinal flow. Magnetic resonance imaging (MRI) studies suggest activity occurs in the endolymphatic sac during attacks of Meniere's disease.[13]

Salt[14] has undertaken some very important work on how endolymph is produced and how it circulates. He has shown that in guinea pigs, the composition of endolymph is maintained by the stria vascularis. The stria vascularis controls the influx of water and modifies the ionic content. Normally there is little flow either radially or longitudinally, and the endolymph is a biologic puddle. If excess endolymph volume occurs, this is reabsorbed back into the stria vascularis (radial flow). Only under exceptional circumstances, such as when there is a large volume increase, does the endolymph move longitudinally to the endolymphatic sac. People can maintain the balance of endolymph by the radial mechanism alone and rarely have to call upon the endolymphatic sac mechanisms to provide longitudinal flow.

The rate of longitudinal flow is restricted by the isthmus of the ED rather like sand draining through an hour glass. It is hypothesized that if the endolymph cannot drain quickly enough, the endolymphatic sinus may act as a reservoir, temporarily holding the excess fluid.

THE IMPORTANCE OF THE UTRICULAR VALVE OF BAST

The purpose of the utricular valve remains debatable. Nevertheless, anatomically, it seems to act as a shutter, so that if longitudinal flow from the cochlea occurs toward the ELS, and endolymph is not drained simultaneously out of the cochlea and semi-circular canals (pars superior) simultaneously.

COCHLEAR FUNCTION BEFORE, DURING, AND AFTER VERTIGO ATTACKS

If a rupture or leakage of potassium through the Reissner membrane occurs, the endo-cochlear potential should crash and cause a severe loss of hearing. To evaluate the cochlear function, patients were supplied with a programmable hearing aid and a portable programmer that allowed them to measure their own hearing.[15] They were asked to measure their pure tone audiometric thresholds daily and if possible during the attacks of vertigo. Six patients were able to measure their hearing during attacks of vertigo, and their hearing thresholds obtained before, during, and after the vertigo attacks were compared. Five of the six subjects showed less than 10 dB hearing level (HL) change in the HLs at all audiometric frequencies before, during, and after the attacks of vertigo. One subject had a probable change in threshold before the attack but not during the attack of vertigo.

Recording of the electrocochleogram during attacks is difficult as the opportunity to test such patients is limited. Furthermore the patient may vomit making it difficult to get stable recordings. The author has succeeded only in two acute case.[16] During the attack little change in the electrocochleogram recordings occurred.

DIRECTION OF THE NYSTAGMUS DURING ACUTE ATTACKS

Nystagmus has been observed during attacks of vertigo, and a horizontal nystagmus is the usual finding. The direction of the nystagmus alters during the course of the attack. The initial direction is subject to some controversy because of the difficulties in observing the patient at this time. Bance and colleagues[17] recorded an attack that began during an electronystagmography session, and they observed an irritative nystagmus for the first 20 seconds, followed by a paralytic nystagmus. Much later in the attack, the nystagmus reverses again, and this is named recovery nystagmus.[18]

THE DRAINAGE THEORY

The drainage theory is a hypothesis that tries to encompass all the previously mentioned aspects of anatomy, physiology, and pathophysiology. The original drainage theory was proposed by Gibson and Arenberg[19] in 1991 but needed modification when it was discovered that longitudinal endolymph flow rarely is needed in people (**Fig. 2**).

A diagram of the membranous labyrinth that emphasizes the various structures is shown in **Fig. 2A**. Excess endolymph volume (endolymphatic hydrops) is shown diagrammatically as a blue color (see **Fig. 2B**). The excess volume tends to accumulate in the apical end of the cochlea, where the membranes are more lax than elsewhere, even though the endolymph pressure would be similar elsewhere in the cochlea. Under normal circumstances, small amounts of excess endolymph can be removed by radial flow, but larger volumes of excess endolymph require longitudinal drainage. Activity in the endolymphatic sac actively draws endolymph toward its lumen (see **Fig. 2C**). When excess endolymph shifts toward the endolymphatic duct, the sinus of the endolymphatic duct can temporarily accommodate any excess that the endo-lymphatic sac is not ready to receive. Usually this excess fluid is removed without any vestibular disturbance, as the endolymphatic valve of Bast helps to isolate the pars superior and prevents endolymph draining out of the utricle.

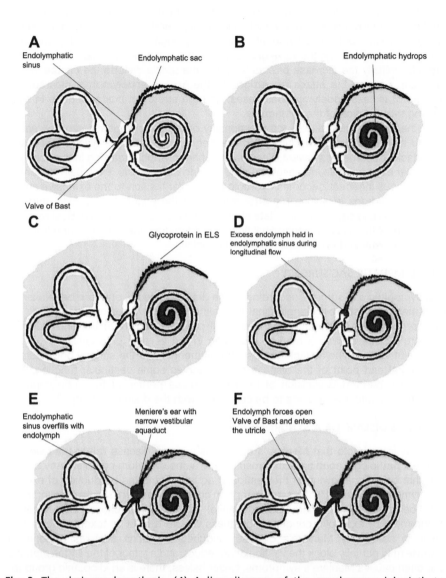

Fig. 2. The drainage hypothesis. (*A*) A line diagram of the membranous labyrinth to emphasize the structures. (*B*) Excess volume of endolymph is illustrated as a blue color in the apical turn. (*C*) The endolymphatic sac secretes and macrophages gobble away the glycoprotein (*green*) to promote longitudinal flow of endolymph. The endolymphatic sinus acts as a reservoir temporarily accommodating endolymph as it trickles through the narrow endolymphatic duct. (*D*) A Meniere's ear has a narrow vestibular duct, and the endolymph trickles more slowly toward the endolymphatic sac. The endolymphatic sinus becomes distended with endolymph. (*E*) The excess endolymph in the endolymphatic sinus forces open the valve of Bast and overflows into the utricle. The increased volume of endolymph in the utricle stretches the cristae of the semicircular canals and causes the attack of vertigo.

If there is a very narrow bony endolymphatic duct limiting the size of the endolymphatic duct, or if debris is partially occluding the duct, endolymph may build up excessively in the sinus of the endolymphatic duct during longitudinal flow (see **Fig. 2**D), and overflow occurs opening the valve of Bast so endolymph enters the pars superior (see **Fig. 2**E). Initially the increase of endolymph in the utricle distorts the cristae in one direction, causing the attack of vertigo. As the excess endolymph is cleared, the amount of excess endolymph decreases, and the stretched cristae reduce in size, altering the direction of the nystagmus.

As the disease progresses, the functionality of the endolymphatic sac decreases due to cellular damage resulting from the frequent secretion of glycoprotein, and the attacks become less severe. The volume of endolymph remaining in the cochlear duct after each episode increases, and the hearing deteriorates. Eventually the entire membranous inner ear becomes hydropic in a similar fashion to the extensive endolymphatic hydrops in guinea pig after removal of the endolymphatic sac, and the attacks of vertigo cease. At these late stages of the disease, the valve of Bast remains patent, and if there is any longitudinal flow, a sudden drainage of endolymph from the utricle will result in drop attacks (Tumarkin attacks).

ENDOLYMPHATIC SAC SURGERY

Endolymphatic sac surgery, according to the drainage theory, only can be explained as a method of stopping longitudinal flow either temporarily or permanently. If the function of the ELS is reduced, the ear will progress rapidly to the end stage of Meniere's disease, with a marked reduction in the severity or a cessation of the attacks of vertigo. The advantage of such treatment is that the surgery only hastens the natural end point of the disease and preserves some vestibular function. The author has performed excision of the extraosseous portion of the endolymphatic sac, and the outcome appears to be consistent with the drainage theory.[20]

MENIERE'S DISEASE OR A SYNDROME?

It seems improbable that Meniere's disease is a single disease rather than several different pathologic conditions that result in the same symptom complex. Any condition that causes narrowing of the vestibular aqueduct and the production of excess endolymph could result in the same symptom complex. The term Meniere's syndrome may be more exact. There are congenital and acquired causes of Meniere's syndrome. For example, congenital deafness due to rubella or toxoplasmosis can result in secondary Meniere's disease; acquired infections such as treponemal disease may partially block the vestibular aqueduct, and a tumor of the endolymphatic sac often causes Meniere's symptoms. Nevertheless, there is an idiopathic group for which no causes have been determined, and perhaps this could be termed Meniere's disease in a similar fashion to the way that Bell palsy has become the term for an idiopathic facial palsy.

Meniere's disease or the idiopathic cause of Meniere's syndrome has a wide spread of the age at onset. The author has analyzed his own series of 1576 patients who had clinically definite Meniere's disease[21] (**Table 1**); the median age is approximately 50 years. This age range is not typical of vascular disorders or autoimmune problems. The age range is somewhat similar to the age of onset of peptic ulcer and gives some support to the notion that Meniere's disease may begin after a viral labyrinthitis in ears that have narrow vestibular aqueducts. The initial episode of viral labyrinthitis causes the endolymphatic hydrops, establishing the syndrome. Perhaps the condition can resolve in the earliest stages after a cluster of attacks. In other

Table 1	
The age at the onset of Meniere's disease (definite category)	
Age at Onset of Symptoms in Years	**Number of Patients**
0–10	1
11–20	16
21–30	96
31–40	221
41–50	393
51–60	380
61–70	310
71–80	137
81–90	22

cases, the viral labyrinthitis may recur and cause another cluster of attacks. Some viruses, such as the herpes virus, may remain in the inner ear, causing several recurrences until eventually the endolymphatic sac functionality is destroyed, causing widespread endolymphatic hydrops similar to the findings after removal of the endolymphatic sac in guinea pigs.[22]

POTENTIAL CAUSES OF EXCESS ENDOLYMPH

Whether the cause of the attacks is due to ruptures, perilymph leakages, or faulty longitudinal drainage, the initiation of individual attacks of vertigo is believed to occur when there is a sudden excess of endolymph. A possible explanation is that there is a critical level that has to be exceeded to cause an attack. If there is an existing excess of endolymph, only a small increase may be required to precipitate an attack of vertigo. Clinicians popularly believe that these small increases could be due to salt retention, hormonal changes, allergies, and even stress. Medical treatment usually is based on these assumptions.

SUMMARY

The wealth of recent research concerning the basic mechanisms of the inner ear casts doubt on the concept of perilymph and endolymph mixing due to ruptures or leakages causing the attacks of vertigo. The structure of the endolymphatic sac has been shown to be complex in people, and an active process is involved in longitudinal drainage of endolymph. The structure of the inner ear seems complex, and the function of the valve of Bast and the endolymphatic sinus is yet to be determined. The homeostasis of endolymph involves ionic replenishment rather than volume changes that longitudinal flow only occurs in response to volume excess. Audiological and electrophysiological studies have revealed little or no change in the cochlear function during episodes of vertigo.

The longitudinal drainage theory hypothesizes that endolymph draining too rapidly from the cochlear duct (pars inferior) causes attacks of vertigo. The endolymph overfills the endolymphatic sinus and overflows into the utricle (pars superior), stretching the cristae of the semicircular canals, causing the attacks.

REFERENCES

1. Ménière P. Mémoire sur des lésions de l'oreille interne donnant lieu à des symptomes cérébrale apoplectiforme. Gaz Méd Paris 1861;16:597–601 [in French].
2. Seymour JC. Vasodilators in the treatment of labyrinthine vascular insufficiencies. J Laryngol Otol 1960;74:133–44.
3. Hallpike CS, Cairns H. Observations on the pathology of Meniere's syndrome. J Laryngol Otol 1938;53:626–55.
4. Yamakawa Y. Über pathologische Veranderung bei einem Meniere Kranken. J Otolaryngol Jpn 1938;44:2310–2 [in German].
5. Schuknecht H. Correlation of pathology with symptoms of Meniere's disease. Otolaryngol Clin North Am 1968;1:433–8.
6. Paparella M, Sajjadi H. The natural history of Meniere's disease. In: Harris JP, editor. Meniere's disease. The Hague (The Netherlands): Kugler Publications; 1999. p. 29–38.
7. Zenner H-P, Ruppersberg JP, Löwenheim H, et al. Pathophysiology: transduction and motor disturbances of hair cells by endolymphatic hydrops and transitory endolymph leakage. In: Harris JP, editor. Meniere's disease. The Hague (The Netherlands): Kugler Publications; 1999. p. 203–17.
8. Lo WM, Daniels DL, Chakeres DW, et al. The endolymphatic sac and duct. AJNR Am J Neuroradiol 1997;18:881–7.
9. Wilbrand HF, Rask-Anderson H, Gilstring D. The vestibular aqueduct and the para-vestibular canal: an anatomic and roentgenologic investigation. Acta Otolaryngol 1974;15:337–55.
10. Rask-Anderson H, Stahle J. Lymphocyte–macrophage activity in the endolymphatic sac: an ultrastructural study of the rugose endolymphatic sac in guinea pig. ORL J Otorhinolaryngol Relat Spec 1979;41:177–92.
11. Lamprecht J, Meyer zum Gottesberge AM. The presence and localization of receptors for atrial natriuretic peptide in the inner ear of the guinea pig. Arch Otorhinolaryngol 1988;45(5):300–1.
12. Rask-Anderson H, Dancckwart-Lilliestrom N, Linthicum FH, et al. Ultrastructural evidence of a merocrine secretion in the human endolymphatic sac. Ann Otol Rhinol Laryngol 1991;100:148–56.
13. Fitzgerald CD, Marks AS. Endolymphatic duct/sac enhancement on gadolinium magnetic resonance imaging of the inner ear: preliminary observations and case reports. Am J Otol 1996;17:603–6.
14. Salt AN. Fluid homeostasis in the inner ear. In: Harris JP, editor. Meniere's disease. The Hague (The Netherlands): Kugler Publications; 1999. p. 93–101.
15. McNeil C, Cohen M, Gibson WPR. Changes in audiometric thresholds before, during and after attacks of vertigo associated with Meniere's syndrome. Acta Otolaryngol 2009;99999:1–4.
16. Gibson WPR. The cause of the attacks of vertigo in Meniere's disease: potassium intoxication theories versus the drainage theory—electrophysiological investigations. In: Lim DJ, editor. 'Meniere's disease & inner ear homeostasis disorders'. Los Angeles (CA): House Ear Institute; 2005. p. 323–4.
17. Bance M, Mai M, Tomlinson D, et al. The changing direction of nystagmus in acute Meniere's disease, pathophysiological implications. Laryngoscope 1991; 101:197–201.
18. Brown DH, McClure JA, Downar-Zapolski Z. The membrane rupture theory of Meniere's disease—is it valid? Laryngoscope 1988;98:599–601.

19. Gibson WPR, Kaufmann Arenberg I. The circulation of endolymph and a new theory of the attacks occurring in Ménière's disease. In: Kaufmann AI, editor. Inner ear surgery. The Hague (The Netherlands): Kugler Publications; 1991. p. 17–23.
20. Gibson WPR. The long term outcome of removal of the endolymphatic sac in Meniere's disease. In: Sterkers O, Ferrary E, Dauman R, et al, editors. Proceedings of the 4th International Ménière's Symposium. New York: Kugler Press; 2000. p. 785–8.
21. Monsell EM, Balkany TM, Gates GA, et al. Committee on hearing and equilibrium guidelines for the diagnosis and evaluation of therapy in Meniere's disease. Otolaryngol Head Neck Surg 1995;113:181–5.
22. Kimura RS. Experimental blockage of the endolymphatic sac and duct and its effect on the inner ear of the guinea pig, a study on endolymphatic hydrops. Ann Otol Rhinol Laryngol 1967;76:664–87.

Premenstrual Exacerbation of Meniere's Disease Revisited

James C. Andrews, MD[a,b,c,]*, Vicente Honrubia, MD, DSc[a,c]

KEYWORDS

• Meniere's disease • Premenstrual • Migraine • Inner ear

A goal of identifying and studying a subpopulation of patients within a disease entity is to better understand the etiology and pathophysiology of the condition so that this information can be applied to the disease in general. Such is the case in Meniere's disease where the subpopulation is identified as those women who have typical symptoms, including ear congestion, fluctuating heaing loss, tinnitus, and crises of vertigo exacerbated during the late luteal phase of the menstrual cycle (premenstrual period).[1]

Menses occurs to prepare the uterus for ovulation.[2] The entire cycle (**Fig. 1**) is dependent on gonadotropic hormones from the anterior pituitary, follicle-stimulating hormone, and luteinizing hormone. The follicular phase of the ovarian cycle occurs with follicle-stimulating hormone acting on the ovum to enlarge and produce various layers, including the theca and granulosa cells, which are primarily responsible for secreting the estrogens and, to a lesser degree, progesterone. Approximately 2 days before ovulation, there is an increase in production of luteinizing hormone, eventually reaching 6 to 10 times its base concentration approximately 18 hours before ovulation. An increase in follicle-stimulating hormone also occurs over this same time period but only increases in 2-fold concentration. The luteinizing hormone causes the theca and granulosa cells to become lutein cells, which secrete progesterone and much less estrogen. There is follicle swelling, degeneration, and rupture that results in release of the ovum. The luteal phase of the ovarian cycle then begins. The remaining theca cells enlarge and undergo luteinization to become the corpus luteum. Once formed, the corpus luteum undergoes a sequential program of proliferation, enlargement, secretion, and degeneration. During its secretory phase, the corpus luteum is producing large amounts of progesterone and estrogen. This

---

[a] Department of Surgery, Northridge Hospital Medical Center, 18350 Roscoe Boulevard, #518, Northridge, CA 91325, USA
[b] Department of Surgery, Sepulveda Veterans Administration Hospital, Sepulveda, CA, USA
[c] David Geffen School of Medicine, UCLA, CA, USA
* Corresponding author. 18350 Roscoe Boulevard, #518, Northridge, CA 91325.
E-mail address: jandrews@mednet.ucla.edu

Otolaryngol Clin N Am 43 (2010) 1029–1040
doi:10.1016/j.otc.2010.05.012
0030-6665/10/$ – see front matter © 2010 Published by Elsevier Inc.

oto.theclinics.com

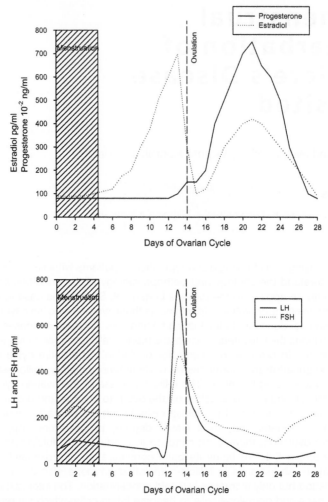

Fig. 1. Plasma concentrations of gonadotropins and ovarian hormones during the normal menstrual cycle.

increase in progesterone and estrogen acts on the anterior pituitary in a feedback mechanism to suppress production of luteinizing and follicle-stimulating hormone. With degeneration of the corpus luteum, there is a drop in progesterone and estrogen levels, which allows for a surge in luteinizing and follicle-stimulating hormone. A new ovarian cycle begins.

REPORT OF A CASE

A 34-year-old woman presented to the authors' clinic with a 7-year history of previously diagnosed Meniere's disease, noting repeated bouts of left-sided hearing loss with documented low-frequency audiometric threshold shifts, low-frequency tinnitus, ear congestion, and sometimes vertigo. The vertigo bouts were severe and could last several hours and usually were associated with nausea and sometimes vomiting. She noted a long history of being treated for migraine headaches with typical aura at their onset, which at times could be associated with her otologic symptoms. She found some relief in lying down in a dark room until they subsided, which required some hours. Approximately 2 years previously she had a period of freedom from symptoms for approximately 15 months from both Meniere's and migraine during and after the pregnancy of her first child, whom she subsequently nursed.

*At the time of her presentation she was on Loestrin 24 (ethinyl estradiol and norethindrone acetate) for birth control and using Diamox (acetazolamide) in attempt to control her Meniere's and migraine symptoms. After trial of various medical regiments, she eventually found success in using a combination of verapamil and Dyazide (triamterene and hydrocholorothiazide) with a low salt diet (<1500 mg sodium per day). She decided to have another child and discontinued her medication although continued with the low salt diet. By having the patient maintain a daily calendar by logging her symptoms and menses, it became notable that her symptoms of unilateral tinnitus and ear congestion were present most of the time but would become more intense during the premenstrual period as would fluctuations in hearing (**Fig. 2**). Some of the premenstrual periods were associated with pronounced episodes of vertigo lasting hours to days. Again, she became pregnant. The tinnitus and congestion continued into the first trimester but hearing fluctuations, vertigo, and headaches improved. The events in this patient are consistent with the putative role of the menstrual cycle in triggering the symptoms of Meniere's disease.*

LITERATURE REVIEW

In 1992, the authors reviewed 109 women with Meniere's disease; 6 were identified with exacerbation of symptoms during the premenstrual period.[1] This was noted by having the patients maintain a calendar and documenting the days of menstrual bleeding as well as symptoms of dizziness, unilateral hearing loss, aural pressure, and tinnitus throughout the month. Although primarily the correlation of the patients' symptoms with the premenstrual period was used to make this diagnosis, serial audiograms were performed showing typical auditory threshold shifts to support this correlation. Within this study, two subgroups of patients could be identified: first, those with early-onset Meniere's disease whose auditory dysfunction was considered reversible, and second, those with long-standing Meniere's disease whose auditory dysfunction was considered irreversible. The patients with reversible disease did not always demonstrate the full spectrum of Meniere's disease initially. Their auditory threshold shifts were considerably more marked and involved all frequencies (**Figs. 2** and **3**). Those with irreversible or long-standing Meniere's disease demonstrated the full spectrum of symptoms all along during the premenstrual period. Their initial auditory thresholds were worse and showed more limited fluctuation.

All patients were managed with a low salt diet and the loop diuretic is triamterene and hydrochlorothiazide (Dyazide). All patients demonstrated control of their vestibular crises symptoms. Those with reversible auditory dysfunction were able to maintain normal hearing. Those with irreversible auditory dysfunction showed stabilization of their hearing but no further improvement. This study again implicates the premenstrual period as an exacerbating factor in the manifestation of symptoms in some women with Meniere's disease.

In another reported study of 5 women with Meniere's disease[3] who could correlate symptoms with their menstrual cycle, two noted their symptoms some days before the menses and three noted their symptoms concomitantly occurred with the menses or immediately thereafter. During pregnancy, vertigo symptoms markedly improved.

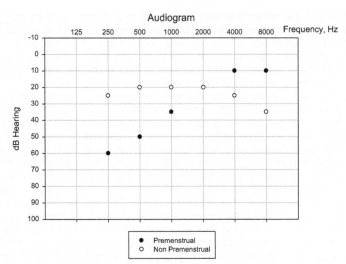

Fig. 2. Audiometric function from the case presentation showing the fluctuation in auditory thresholds when the patient noted hearing loss during the premenstrual period. This is compared with when the patient noted no hearing loss during the nonpremenstrual state.

After the pregnancy, some patients noted the return of Meniere's symptoms with their menstrual cycle. With interruption of the menstrual cycles by pregnancy, there was improvement in the Meniere's symptoms, only to have them return after childbirth. This report provides further evidence of the premenstrual period as the aggravating factor in this group of Meniere's patients.

In an Internet-based research study, subjects with Meniere's disease were recruited from a website.[4] In the first phase of the study, 42 women with purported Meniere's disease were identified that could correlate the symptoms of their condition with the menstrual cycle. In the second phase of the study, 20 women were invited to participate by maintaining calendars and filling out questionnaires to assess their condition on a daily basis. They were compared with 17 men with Meniere's disease as a control. In the third phase of the study, the female subjects were asked to use over-the-counter urinary ovulation kits, which were then returned by mail to the investigators to analyze more specifically the timing of ovulation to compare with their reported symptoms. Eleven women were able to complete the study. Vertigo was noted as the significant symptom that would diminish post menses in those women with premenstrual exacerbation of Meniere's disease.

There are several additional case reports regarding premenstrual symptoms of fluctuating hearing loss, tinnitus, and vertigo.[1,5,6] In some of these reports, symptoms develop bilaterally.[7] In others, symptoms are unilateral and exacerbated during the premenstrual period.

Price and colleagues[8] describe a patient with Meniere's disease exacerbated during the luteal phase of the menstrual cycle. The patient's symptoms were completely controlled using leuprolide acetate (a gonadotropin-releasing hormone) but returned on cessation of treatment. Andreyko and Jaffe[9] described a patient with a 40-dB auditory threshold fluctuation, which always occurred in the luteal phase of her menstrual cycle. Similarly, her symptoms were completely controlled with nafarelin (a gonadotropin-releasing hormonal agonist) only to return after the cessation of this medication. The use of gonadotropin-releasing hormones is to bind to the pituitary gonadotropin-releasing hormone receptors and suppress gonadotropin secretion,

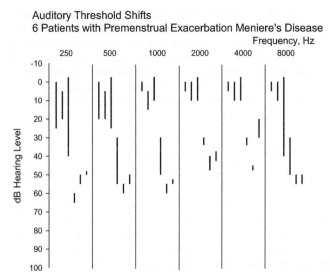

Fig. 3. Auditory threshold shifts in six women with Meniere's disease during the premenstrual period. For each frequency there are six high-low lines (one for each patient) showing the shift in threshold from the premenstrual to the nonpremenstrual period. The top of each bar represents the patients' better audiometric function during the nonpremenstrual period. The bottom of the bar represents the patients' poorer audiometric function during the premenstrual period. The first three patients in each frequency are those with reversible Meniere's disease and show the more marked fluctuation in threshold, involve all the tested frequencies and considerably better outcome. The second three patients are those with irreversible Meniere's disease and show less fluctuation in threshold and poorer eventual outcome. (*Data from* Andrews J, Ator GA, Honrubia V. The exacerbation of symptoms in Meniere's disease during the premenstrual period. Arch Otolaryngol Head Neck Surg 1992;118:74–8.)

resulting in the cessation of ovulation. With complete interruption of the menstrual cycle, these patients' disease was controlled. Together, all these reports corroborate that the fundamental pathology of the inner ear symptoms were associated with the premenstrual period.

DISCUSSION

Stress as an emotional, mental, or physical condition has been considered an exacerbating factor that produces crises symptoms in Meniere's patients within a period of hours.[7,10] Psychological stress, plasma levels of antidiuretic hormone, and exacerbation of symptoms in Meniere's disease were correlated in another study.[11] It has been recognized that in some women with Meniere's disease, this stress condition can be the premenstrual period.[1]

Understanding the instability of the inner ear that can produce the symptoms of Meniere's disease and then recover to become asymptomatic has been a continued challenge. Although it is well considered that the morphologic changes of endolymphatic hydrops are not always correlated to the inner ear symptoms produced in Meniere's disease.[12,13] The pathologic state exists and in some patients can be very symptomatic. The concept of the Meniere's inner ear being in a functional yet volatile state, which can be triggered by additional force or stress to produce symptoms, is appealing.

A point of consideration is that the reported cases of premenstrual exacerbation of Meniere's disease have largely been reported as a unilateral affliction of the inner ear. Yet the hormonal and bodily mechanisms that are considered exacerbating factors should involve the entire body or organism. There lacks a logical explanation for this unilateral inner ear dysfunction other than one ear may be more predisposed to Meniere's disease over the other. This is an area that requires more investigation. Other mechanisms associated with the pathophysiology of the condition are being investigated and are described later.

HORMONES, WATER RETENTION, AND FLUID SHIFTS

Commonly noted by many women during the premenstrual period are weight gain and body water redistribution or fluid shift. In metabolically controlled conditions, women can gain up to 1 kg of weight during this time.[14] Not all women gain weight yet they describe a sensation of being bloated or swollen during this time. Alterations in the capillary wall integrity to water may allow for a vascular fluid shift to the interstitial compartment.[15,16] An increase in the capillary coefficient of 30% has been demonstrated.[15] MRI studies have shown shifts in cerebrospinal fluid volume of up 13.4% during the premenstrual period.[17] Increase in the intraocular pressure in women with glaucoma during the premenstrual period has been noted as well.[18]

The extrauterine effects of estrogen and especially progesterone on water and electrolyte balance can be substantial. Similar in chemical structure to aldosterone, these hormones can cause sodium and water reabsorbtion from the distal tubule of the kidney.[2] An increase in aldosterone as well as possibly vasopressin can occur during the premenstrual period. The net effect is reabsorbtion of sodium from the distal tubule and an increase in sodium in the extracellular tissues. Hypernatremia is not noted in that usually an increase in thirst and water intake acts to dilute the sodium that is absorbed. Estrogen and progesterone can also produce glucocorticoid results similar to cortisol including fluid retention.

The handling of sodium load by the body is different during the phases of the menstrual cycle.[19] In the luteal phase, sodium intake causes renal vasodilation and a reduced filtration fraction. Largely there is retention of sodium from the distal nephron. The net effect is to retain fluid. In the follicular phase, sodium intake causes no renal vascular effect and a decrease in sodium reabsorbtion from the proximal and distal tubule of the kidney. The cause of this variance in sodium handling has been considered secondary to the serum estrogen, and possibly progesterone levels, which may modulate the renal hydrodynamics. In another study of normal premenstrual women, a sodium restricted diet (<1600 mg of sodium per day) could significantly alter extracellular fluid volume and sodium balance during the luteal phase.[20] The importance of these differences in sodium handling in various phases of the menstrual cycle has important ramifications in the success of a low salt diet to manage symptoms especially during the premenstrual period. It is also important to note that the same sodium restriction in the follicular phase of the cycle is less likely to have such an effect.

The premenstrual syndrome and a particularly more severe form, the premenstrual dysphoric disorder, are specific conditions that occur in the late luteal phase but up to 2 weeks before the onset of the menses and accompanied by relief of symptoms thereafter. Symptoms include depression, angry outbursts, irritability, anxiety, confusion, breast tenderness, abdominal bloating, headache, and swelling of extremeties. The number of symptoms, severity, and frequency of occurrence with the menses can differentiate the syndrome from the dysphoric disorder. These conditions have been correlated with excessive levels of aldosterone and antidiuretic hormone.

Nonpharmalogic treatment can often be successful, which typically includes dietary sodium restriction. For the severe premenstrual syndrome and the dysphoric disorder that does not respond to simple measures, phamacologic treatment can include agents that increase central nervous system serotonin levels. These conditions can be alleviated by interruption of the menstrual cycle and are, therefore, are considered to be hormonal.[21,22]

The aquaporin system becomes an attractive consideration in the possible development and manifestation of Meniere's disease from the vantage point of a hormonal fluid balance disorder. The discovery of these ubiquitous channels that actively move water within bodily spaces and compartments could well be involved and are being investigated in several laboratories. Antidiuretic hormone (also known as vasopressin) works on the vasopressin-2 receptors to activate the aquaporin-2 channels, which in turn moves water from the kidneys tubular lumen into the cell. Within the inner ear, aquaporin-2 receptors have been found with a high concentration in the endolymphatic sac in the human and guinea pig as well as the stria vascularis of the rat.[23] For some time a correlation between antidiuretic hormone and exacerbation of Meniere's disease has been proposed. Several studies have investigated serum concentrations of antidiuretic hormone with patients with Meniere's disease with inconclusive results. Lim and colleagues[24] found no significant correlation of antidiuretic hormone serum levels with unilateral disease. Aoki and colleagues[25] showed that during Meniere's crises that there was an increase in antidiuretic hormone concentration. Meniere's disease was reported in two patients (twins) with congenital nephrogenic diabetes insipidus compensatory to high levels of antidiuretic hormone.[26] Kitahara and colleagues[27] took a different approach by measuring the concentration of vasopressin-2 receptor sites in endolymphatic sac specimens from patients undergoing sac surgery for Meniere's disease. They compared the concentration of vasopressin-2 receptor sites in patients undergoing acoustic neuroma surgery and were able to show significantly greater concentration of vasopressin-2 receptor sites in the Meniere's group. The indication is that the number of available vasopressin-2 receptor sites available in the affected ear may be more important than the serum level of antidiuretic hormone in producing Meniere's disease. Other aquaporin channels have been identified as well, including aquaporin-1 in most of the inner ear, aquaporin-4 in the supporting cells of the cochlea and vestibular end organs, and aquaporin-5 in the organ of Corti and Reissner membrane.[28]

A pioneer animal laboratory study by Bosher and Warren[29] was of relevance to the problem of premenstrual exacerbation of Meniere's disease. In part of their study, they looked at the inner ear effect of systemic administration of a hypo-osmotic agent. Distilled water injected intraperitoneally could significantly decrease the osmotic pressure of the endolymph and perilymph within a period of 26 minutes and subsequently show recovery to near normal within 2 hours. Corresponding intralabyrinthine changes resulting in an increase in osmotic pressure were noted with systemic administration of hyperosmolar agents. At the time, the investigators conjectured that some portion of the membranes bounding the endolymphatic space to be near freely permeable to water.

The question arises as to how the premenstrual period exacerbates crises symptoms in a patient with Meniere's disease. The hormonal effects of the premenstrual period result in sodium and water retention by the kidney, which affects the entire body. The inner ear may respond with an increase in osmotic as well as intralabyrinthine pressure. A differential increase in endolymphatic over perilymphatic pressure would result in outward displacement of the basilar membrane. This subsequently may result in distortion of movement of the organ of Corti during acoustic stimulation.[30] Similar endolymphatic pressure increase in the labyrinth would alter motion of the cupula during angular rotation. Increased intralabyrinthine pressure could potentially affect blood circulation within the stria vascularis, especially the venules and capillaries. A relative increase in endolymph sodium and concomitant decrease in potassium combined with circulatory changes could lead to a decrease in endococlear potential. The resulting effect would be a decrease in excitability of the hair cell neural complex with decreased spontaneous activity, increased thresholds of stimulation, and diminished response.

OTHER POTENTIAL MECHANISMS

A causative factor of the premenstrual syndrome in some women has been shown to be hypothyroidism. In these women, supplemental thyroid has been successful in their treatment.[31,32] A correlation of thyroid dysfunction in patients with Meniere's disease has also been shown. Brenner and colleagues[33] showed that 32% of patients with Meniere's disease were being concomitantly treated with supplemental thyroid. Of the Meniere's patients Fattori and colleagues[34] studied, 14% were hypothyroid and 38% showed the presence of thyroid autoantibodies, which was highly significant.

A significant increase in blood viscosity occurs in many women during the premenstrual period, the mechanism of which remains unknown.[35,36] Clinically as well as experimentally, the effect of an increase in blood viscosity has the greatest effect on the small blood vessels. The inner ear, being a microvascular end organ without collateral blood flow, is extremely vulnerable to such a condition. It has been previously reported that increased blood viscosity can result in inner ear dysfunction with symptoms of hearing loss, tinnitus, and vertigo.[37]

MENIERE'S DISEASE, MIGRAINE, AND THE PREMENSTRUAL PERIOD

Meniere's disease, migraine, and the premenstrual period become a difficult quandary. Migrainous vertigo can appear similar to Meniere's disease with vertiginous crises episodes, durations, and associated symptoms of hearing loss, tinnitus, and aural fullness.[38,39] Half the patients with migrainous vertigo do not have headaches at the time of vestibular dysfunction. It has been that suggested migrainous vertigo may be ear related and secondary to vasospasm or defective ion channel.[40] Some investigators propose that the progressive hearing loss characteristic of Meniere's disease does not occur in migraine.[41] Whether or not to include or exclude patients with a history of migraine headache may be a matter of semantics. An epidemiologic study did not show an increased incidence of migraine headache in patients with Meniere's disease.[42] Adding the potential of premenstrual exacerbation into consideration makes the matter more complex. It is well documented that the premenstrual period can act as a trigger for migraine and some studies estimate that up to 60% of premenopausal women with migraine have an association with the menstrual cycle.[43,44] It may be surmised that the premenstrual period may also trigger migrainous vertigo. Migraine may trigger a Meniere's crisis, perhaps by acting on an underlying pathologic ear. Decline in estrogen levels in the late luteal phase of the menstrual cycle is considered the actual hormonal manipulation that triggers the migraine.[45] Research as to the potential of aquaporins related to migraine is being considered as well.[46,47]

TREATMENT

Management of patients with premenstrual exacerbation remains similar in general to that of patients with Meniere's disease. A low salt diet and a loop diuretic, such as

Dyazide or Maxide, are effective. Having patients maintain a daily calendar can be helpful in understanding not only the physiology of the disease but also its management. When the symptoms are likely to occur, it can be useful to diligently control sodium intake or to increase the diuretic dose. Some patients are managed with a low salt diet until a few days before the premenstrual period when a diuretic is added. Patients have to be educated as to their condition and have the intelligence to self-medicate. Oral contraceptives are an option as well, although it is variable as to whether or not patients respond to this treatment. Based on the authors' previous clinical experience, these patients responded well to medical and dietary management. Most important, given the reversibility of the condition in the majority of the patients, ablative procedures, such as intratympanic injections of aminoglycosides, should not be considered as a first-line treatment. Complete interruption of the menstrual cycle, although effective, cannot be used for more than a few months because of long-term hormonal complications. If migraine is a factor, oral contraceptives can be helpful with the use of a prophylactic migraine medication (β-blocker or calcium channel blocker) with an increase in the dosage during the premenstrual period.[45,48–50]

MECHANISM OF TREATMENT

Within the inner ear, the endocochlear potential is regarded as produced and maintained by the stria vascularis.[51] There are several potassium channels important in maintaining the high potassium gradient between the endolymph and perilymph as well as between the endolymph and the blood and interstitial fluid. Some of these potassium channels are responsible for the positive endocochlear potential whereas others maintain the gradient and additionally are important in the production of endolymph.[52] Potassium channels are located in the marginal cells, intermediate cells, and fibrocytes as well as the dark cells of the vestibular labyrinth. There is a flow of potassium within the cochlea through the sensory cells toward the spiral ligament.[52] One mechanism proposed that the perilymph released by the hair cells is recycled through the supporting cells by way of a gap junction system.[53] Earlier work by Bosher[54] on ethacrynic acid and and by Pike and Bosher[55] on furosemide indicates that these loop diuretics affect the potassium concentration of the endolymph and subsequently the endocochlear potential. It is likely that the clinically useful hydrochlorothiazide/triamterene loop diuretic affects the potassium channels of the cochlea and vestibular labyrinth. The effect may be to (1) reduce endolymph production and (2) reduce the endocochlear potential and sensitivity of the inner ear, which subsequently would reduce vestibular instability and crises of vertigo. Additionally, a low salt diet and a diuretic are effective in reducing the hydration of the overall individual. This in turn may have a beneficial effect on the inner ear.

SUMMARY

Some women with Meniere's disease demonstrate exacerbation of symptoms during the premenstrual period. It is believed that the hormonal stress of the premenstrual period acts on the volatile inner ear with Meniere's disease to result in dysfunction. The hormonal effects of the premenstrual period include alterations in sodium and water balance through changes in plasma estrogen, progesterone, aldosterone, and antidiuretic hormone. These hormonal effects are likely to influence the aquaporin system. Other physiologic alterations of the premenstrual period that can affect the inner ear include changes in thyroid hormone levels and blood viscosity. Migraine, Meniere's disease, and the premenstrual period may be a complex interaction leading to exacerbation of symptoms. Having patients maintain a daily calendar of symptoms, diet, and menses can be helpful in understanding the disease as well as instigating treatment monitoring. Most patients can be effectively managed with dietary sodium restriction and a loop diuretic.

REFERENCES

1. Andrews J, Ator GA, Honrubia V. The exacerbation of symptoms in Meniere's disease during the premenstrual period. Arch Otolaryngol Head Neck Surg 1992;118:74–8.
2. Guyton AC. Textbook of medical physiology. Philadelphia: W.B. Saunders Co; 1976. p. 1086–103.
3. Watanabe I, Imai S, Ikeda M, et al. Meniere's disease and the menstrual cycle. In: Sterkers O, Ferrary E, Sauvage JP, et al, editors. Meniere's disease 1999—update. Netherlands: Kugler Publ; 1999. p. 463–6.
4. Morse GG, House JW. Changes in Meniere's disease responses as a function of the menstrual cycle. Nurs Res 2001;5:286–92.
5. Miller MH, Gould WJ. Fluctuating sensorineural hearing impairment associated with the menstrual cycle. J Aud Res 1967;7:373–85.
6. Souaid J, Rappaport JM. Fluctuating sensorineural hearing loss associated with the menstrual cycle. J Otolaryngol 2000;30:246–50.
7. Al-Mana D, Ceranic B, Djahanbakhch O, et al. Hormones and the auditory system: a review of physiology and pathophysiology. Neuroscience 2008;153: 881–900.
8. Price TM, Allen TC, Bowyer DL, et al. Ablation of luteal phase symptoms of Meniere's disease with leuprolide. Arch Otolaryngol 1994;120:209–11.
9. Andreyko JL, Jaffe RB. Use of a gonadotropin-releasing hormone agonist analogue for of cyclic auditory dysfunction. Obstet Gynecol 1989;74(3Pt 2):506–9.
10. Hessen Soderman AC, Moller J, Bagger-Sjoback D, et al. Stress as a trigger of attacks in Meniere's disease. A case-crossover study. Laryngoscope 2004;114: 1843–8.
11. Sawada S, Takeda T, Saito H. Antidiuretic hormone and psychosomatic aspects in Meniere's disease. Acta Otolaryngol Suppl 1997;528:109–12.
12. Merchant SN, Adams JC, Nadol JB. Pathophysiology of Meniere's syndrome: are symptoms caused by endolymphatic hydrops? Otol Neurotol 2005;26:74–81.
13. Rauch SD, Merchant SN, Thedinger BA. Meniere's syndrome and endolymphatic hydrops: double-blind temporal bone study. Ann Otol Rhinol Laryngol 1989;98: 873–83.
14. Friederich MA. Psychophysiology of menstruation and the menopause. In: Romney SI, Gray MJ, Little AB, et al, editors. Gynecology and obstetrics: the health care of women. New York: McGraw-Hill Book Co; 1975. p. 603–15 Chapter 34.
15. Tollan A, Oian P, Fadnes HO, et al. Evidence for altered transcapillary fluid balance in women with the premenstrual syndrome. Acta Obstet Gynecol Scand 1993;72:238–42.
16. Wong WH, Freedman RI, Levan NE, et al. Changes in the capillary filtration of cutaneous vessels in women with premenstrual tension. Br J Obstet Gynaecol 1972;114:950–3.
17. Grant R, Condon B, Lawrence A. Is cranial CSF volume under hormonal influence? An MR study. J Comput Assist Tomogr 1988;12:36–9.
18. Dalton K. Influence of menstruation on glaucoma. Br J Ophthalmol 1967;51: 692–5.

19. Pechere-Bertschi A, Maillard M, Stalder H, et al. Renal segment tubular response to salt during the normal menstrual cycle. Kidney Int 2002;61:425–31.
20. Olson BR, Forman M, Lanza E, et al. Relation between sodium balance and menstrual cycle symptoms in normal women. Ann Intern Med 1996;125:564–7.
21. Watts JF. Hormonal studies in women with premenstrual tension. Br J Obstet Gynaecol 2005;92:247–55.
22. Gray MJ, Strausfield KS, Watanabe M, et al. Aldosterone secretory rates in the normal menstrual cycle. J Clin Endocrinol 1969;28:1269–75.
23. Couloigner V, Berrebi D, Teixeira M, et al. Aquaporin-2 in the human endolymphatic sac. Acta Otolaryngol 2004;124:449–53.
24. Lim JS, Lange ME, Megerian CA. Serum antidiuretic hormone levels in patients with unilateral Meniere's disease. Laryngoscope 2003;113:1321–6.
25. Aoki M, Ando K, Kuze B, et al. The association of antidiuretic hormone levels with an attack of Meniere's disease. Clin Otolaryngol 2005;30:521–55.
26. Commacchio F, Boggian O, Poletta E, et al. Meniere's disease in congenital nephrogenic diabetes insipidus: report of two twins. Am J Otol 1992;13:477–81.
27. Kitahara T, Doi C, Maekawa C, et al. Meniere's attacks occur in the inner ear with excessive vasopressin type-2 receptors. J Neuroendocrinol 2008;20:1295–300.
28. Beitz E, Zenner HP, Schultz JE. Aquaporin-mediated fluid regulation in the inner ear. Cell Mol Neurobiol 2003;23:315–29.
29. Bosher SK, Warren RL. A study of the electrochemistry and osmotic relationships of the cochlear fluids in the neonatal rat at the time of of the development of the endocochlear potential. J Physiol 1971;212:739–61.
30. Honrubia V. Pathophysiology of Meniere's disease: vestibular system. In: Harris JP, editor. Meniere's disease. Netherlands: Kugler Publ; 1999. p. 231–60.
31. Brayshaw ND, Brayshaw DD. Thyroid hypofunction in the premenstrual syndrome. N Engl J Med 1986;315:1486–7.
32. Schmit PJ, Khan RA, Rubinow DR. Thyroid function in premenstrual syndrome. N Engl J Med 1987;317:1537–8.
33. Brenner M, Hofstad DL, Hain TC. Prevalence of thyroid dysfunction in patients with Meniere's disease. Arch Otolaryngol Head Neck Surg 2004;130:226–8.
34. Fattori B, Nacci A, Dardano A, et al. Possible association between thyroid autoimmunity and Meniere's disease. Clin Exp Immunol 2008;152:28–32.
35. Simpson LO. The etiopathogenesis of the premenstrual syndrome as a consequence of altered blood rheology. Med Hypotheses 1988;25:189–95.
36. Dintenfass L, Julian DG, Miller G. Viscosity of blood in healthy young women: effect of the premenstrual cycle. Lancet 1966;1:234.
37. Andrews JC, Hoover LA, Lee RS, et al. Vertigo in the hyperviscosity syndrome. Otolaryngol Head Neck Surg 1988;98:144–9.
38. Furman JM, Marcus DA, Balaban CD. Migrainous vertigo: development of a pathogenetic model and structured diagnostic interview. Curr Opin Neurol 2003;16:5–13.
39. Neuheauser H, Lempert T. Vertigo and dizziness related to migraine: a diagnostic challenge. Cephalalgia 2004;24:83–91.
40. Brantberg K, Trees N, Baloh RW. Migraine-associated vertigo. Acta Otolaryngol 2005;125:276–9.
41. von Brevern M, Zeise D, Neuhauser H, et al. Acute migrainous vertigo: clinical and oculographic findings. Brain 2005;128:365–74.
42. Gopen Q, Viire E, Anderson J. Epidemiologic study to explore links between Meniere's syndrome and migraine headache. Ear Nose Throat J 2009;88:1200–4.

43. Landy S. Migraine throughout the life cycle: treatment through the ages. Neurology 2004;62(Suppl 2):S2–8.
44. Calhoun AH. A novel specific prophylaxis for menstrual-associated migraine. South Med J 2004;97:819–22.
45. Tozer BS, Boatwright EA, David PS, et al. Prevention of migraine in women throughout the life span. Mayo Clin Proc 2006;81:1086–92.
46. Wakayama Y, Inoue M, Takahashi J. Aquaporin-1 may be involved in the pathophysiology of migraine: a hypothesis. Headache 2007;47:1457–8.
47. Rainero RE, Crasto VG, Brega NE, et al. Investigating the genetic role of aquaporin-4 gene in migraine. J Headache Pain 2009;10:111–4.
48. Massiou H, MacGregor EA. Evolution and treatment of migraine with oral contraceptives. Cephalalgia 2000;20:170–4.
49. Martin VT, Lipton RB. Epidemiology and biology of menstrual migraine. Headache 2008;48(Suppl 3):5124–30.
50. Seemungal BM, Gresty MA, Bronstein AM. The endocrine system, vertigo and balance. Curr Opin Neurol 2001;14:27–34.
51. von Bekesy G. DC potentials and energy balance of the cochlear partion. J Acoust Soc Am 1950;22:576–82.
52. Wangemann P. K^+ cycling and the endocochlear potential. Hear Res 2002;165:1–9.
53. Spicer SS, Schulte BA. The fine structure of spiral ligament cells realtes to ion return to the stria and vearies with place-frequency. Hear Res 1996;100:80–100.
54. Bosher SK. The nature of the negative endocochlear potentials produced by anoxia and ethacrynic acid in the rat and guinea pig. J Physiol 1979;293:329–45.
55. Pike DA, Bosher SK. The time course of the strial changes produced by intravenous furosemide. Hear Res 1980;3:79–89.

Meniere's Disease in the Elderly

Dominique Vibert, MD*, Marco Caversaccio, MD,
Rudolf Häusler, MD

KEYWORDS

- Elderly • Meniere's disease • Drop attacks • Otolith organs
- Endolymphatic hydrops

Dizziness and vertigo are common complaints in the elderly population. However, these symptoms may be a result of multiple causes, such as cardiovascular disease, secondary effects of medication, and pathologies of the central nervous system, as well as inner ear diseases.

Among a population of 3427 patients 70 years of age or older, Katsarkas[1] found that 55.30% of them suffered from vertigo caused by an inner ear disease such as positional vertigo (47.20%), vestibular neuronitis (4.07%), and Meniere's disease (4.07%).

The typical criteria of Meniere's disease include the onset of recurrent attacks of vertigo lasting for a few hours with nausea and vomiting. The patients also complain of fluctuating hearing loss, an intermittent sensation of fullness, and a transient or permanent tinnitus within the impaired ear. Drop attacks, consisting of sudden falls without loss of consciousness, first described by Tumarkin,[2] can also occur in patients suffering from Meniere's disease. They are attributed to a sudden dysfunction of the otolithic organs and are also named "otolithic catastrophe of Tumarkin." Depending on the studies, the incidence of Meniere's disease ranges from 10 to 1000 per 100,000 patients of the ear, nose, and throat population.[3–6]

Meniere's disease usually begins in adults ranging in age from 20 to 60 years.[7–9] It is rarely described in children, who represent about 1% of Meniere's patients.[4,10–14] However, that the real incidence of Meniere's disease focuses on older patients was first reported by Ballester and colleagues.[6] They found that among 432 patients suffering from Meniere's disease, 15.3% were 65 years or older. In a recent retrospective study about the origin of vertigo and dizziness in 677 patients older than 65, Üneri and Polat[15] found a similar percentage of 12.5% of patients suffering from Meniere's disease. These 2 studies tend to demonstrate that Meniere's disease occurs more

Department of Otorhinolaryngology, Head and Neck Surgery, Inselspital, University of Berne, 3010 Berne, Switzerland
* Corresponding author. Neurotology, University Clinic of ENT, Head and Neck Surgery Inselspital, 3010 Berne, Switzerland.
E-mail address: dominique.vibert@insel.ch

Otolaryngol Clin N Am 43 (2010) 1041–1046
doi:10.1016/j.otc.2010.05.009
0030-6665/10/$ – see front matter © 2010 Elsevier Inc. All rights reserved.

oto.theclinics.com

frequently than previously thought in patients older than 65. Although it seems that both sexes are almost equally affected in adult patients,[8] Ballester and colleagues[6] described a strong preponderance in women, with a sex ratio of 0.43 in their patients. This sex preponderance was also reported in the study of Üneri and Polat.[15] That women are more afflicted in this age range might be directly related to their longer life span compared with that of men. Ballester and colleagues[6] distinguished 2 different groups of patients in their study. One group of patients from 65 to 75 years suffered from a reactivation of longstanding Meniere's disease, which represented 40.9% of the cohort, and a second group of patients demonstrated the first manifestations of Meniere's disease occurring between the ages of 65 and 82 years. The percentage of this "de novo" Meniere's disease reaches 59.1% of all patients. In both groups, the clinical manifestations were similar to the classic vertigo spells lasting from minutes to hours, with nausea and sometimes with vomiting as well as the sensorineural hearing loss with fluctuation of hearing and tinnitus. However, the drop attacks were more frequent in the "de novo" group, occurring in 25.6% of patients compared with 11.1% in patients with a reactivation of their longstanding Meniere's disease. This study underlined 2 interesting facts: the preponderance of women and the high frequency of drop attacks in patients older than 65.

In the general population of Meniere's disease with patients younger than 65 years, the incidence of drop attacks varies between 5% and 10%[16–18]; however, Kentala and colleagues[19] reported an extremely high incidence of drop attacks in 72% of their patients with Meniere's disease aged from 17 to 79 years. In this study, the mean age at onset of the disease was 44 years, and they classified the drop attacks in 3 degrees (mild, moderate, severe) depending on the ensuing daily disturbances. Nine percent of the patients suffered severe disturbances. This percentage is therefore consistent with those in the literature with studies performed in the general population of patients with Meniere's disease. Kentala and colleagues[19] explained this high prevalence of drop attacks was because patients would probably not have spontaneously reported that the drop attacks caused mild or moderate disability if they had not been specifically asked. Thus, compared with the literature data, the group of patients with "de novo" Meniere's disease in the elderly population showed a higher incidence of 25.6% of drop attacks.

Feelings of erroneous movements such as the sensation of being pushed from behind or of a sudden movement of the environment are frequently described by patients with drop attacks. These symptoms are attributed to a dysfunction of the otolithic organs that measure the linear accelerations in the horizontal and vertical axes as well as the gravitational vector. Several pathophysiological mechanisms are thought to be implicated in the otolithic catastrophe of Tumarkin: sudden shift of the utricular macula, sudden changes in the endolymphatic fluid pressure, and sudden electrolyte changes secondary to the rupture of the membrane labyrinth. Thus, the inappropriate stimulation of the otolithic organs might generate a failure of the vestibulospinal reflex with the loss of postural tonus and, consequently, the falling.[16,19–22] To explain the higher incidence of drop attacks, particularly in patients with "de novo" Meniere's disease, Ballester and colleagues[6] assumed that it could be linked to a decreased compliance of the otolithic structures with a lower tolerance of the hydrops, owing to a limited capacity of the endolymphatic compartment distension. They also took into account the progressive decline of postural control and gait and visual difficulties of the elderly as factors able to influence the onset of falls.

However, based on several recently published articles, new hypotheses might be proposed to explain these 2 characteristics within this specific population of patients, ie, the high incidence of drop attacks and the prevalence in women.

ON THE COCHLEAR SIDE

On review of 107 archival temporal bone cases with the clinical diagnosis of Meniere's disease or the histopathologic diagnosis of hydrops, Merchant and colleagues[23] suggested that endolymphatic hydrops must be considered as an epiphenomenon of Meniere's disease rather than being directly its cause. They considered that hydrops should be a marker for disordered homeostasis of the labyrinth. Indeed, Ichimiya and colleagues,[24] Nadol and colleagues,[25] and Shinomori and colleagues[26] demonstrated cytochemical changes and ultrastructural lesions within type I and type II fibrocytes of the spiral ligament in experimental endolymphatic hydrops. They are involved in the recycling of K^+ ions within the scala media.[27,28] Furthermore, the role of calcium homeostasis implicated in endolymphatic hydrops has been suspected for several decades.[29–31]

Several studies have shown that an induced endolymphatic hydrops in guinea pigs generated a number of biochemical changes,[25] and particularly a marked decrease of immunoreactivity in calcium-binding proteins such as calmodulin, caldesmon, osteopontin, and S-100 among the type I fibrocytes.[24] It was also suggested that the dysfunction of type I fibrocytes may be involved in regulating Ca++ levels in cochlear fluids.[24]

ON THE VESTIBULAR SIDE

Several experimental studies demonstrated the presence of calcium at all levels of the ultrastructure of the otolithic organs.[32–36] These findings pointed out the important role that calcium plays in the otolithic organs and their function. The recurrent benign paroxysmal positional vertigo, attributed to a dysfunction of the otolithic organs, was suspected to be related to a disturbance of calcium metabolism such as osteoporosis/osteopenia in women older than 50.[37] This hypothesis was then corroborated by the results of an experimental study performed in female adult rats showing ultrastructural changes on the utricles of the osteoporotic rats, in terms of size and density, as well as aspect of otoconia.[38]

Thus, the high incidence of "de novo" Meniere's disease as well as the high incidence in women and drop attacks in patients aged 65 or older might be related to the specific impact of the role of calcium metabolism in the elderly. Furthermore, drop attacks seem to occur more frequently in women than men (Dominique Vibert personal unpublished data, 2009). Thus, this difference might be because the disturbances of calcium metabolism that generate osteopenia or osteoporosis are more predominant in postmenopausal women compared with men.

The treatment of Meniere's disease in the elderly represents a challenge because of the polymedication that is very often administered for other concomitant systemic diseases. On one hand, in most cases, antivertiginous drugs such as betahistine and cinnarizin give good results with minor secondary effects. On the other hand, neuroleptics and antihistaminics are more difficult to administer because of their side effects, such as parkinsonism and depression, particularly in cases of long-term treatment.

Chemical labyrinthectomy, by instillation of gentamycin into the middle ear, can also be proposed,[39–41] but unfavorable evolution with incapacitating ataxia may sometimes be observed.[6]

Minor surgical procedures such as insertion of transtympanic ventilation tubes and transcanalar sacculotomy are reported as to be effective and suppress the vertigo attacks in more than 70% of cases.[6,42–44] Nevertheless, sacculotomy represents a risk, with profound postoperative hearing loss reported in 10% to 20% of cases.[43,45]

Definitive vestibular surgical deafferentations, such as labyrinthectomy and selective vestibular neurectomy, represent optional procedures but must be carefully evaluated from case to case for patients with intractable recurrent attacks of vertigo resistant to other treatments. Ablative procedures remain the efficient treatment of drop attacks, taking into account the potential risks of severe injuries occurring in cases of sudden falls. When the general physical condition of the patient is good without comorbidity, such as sensory ataxia, cerebellar dysfunction, and poor vision, older patients are able to satisfactorily compensate the peripheral vestibular deafferentation.[6,46–49]

SUMMARY

Meniere's disease occurs more frequently than previously thought in patients older than 65 years. Two different groups of patients are distinguishable: patients with reactivation of a longstanding Meniere's disease and patients with "de novo" disease.

Compared with general Meniere's patients, this specific population shows a high incidence of women as well as a high incidence of drop attacks, especially among patients with "de novo" Meniere's disease.

Because of the even lengthier life span of the occidental population, the potential risks of severe injuries caused by the drop attacks and their social consequences might represent a real problem for public health in terms of suitable care proposed to these patients.

REFERENCES

1. Katsarkas A. Dizziness in aging: the clinical experience. Geriatrics 2008;63(11): 18–20.
2. Tumarkin A. The otolithic catastrophe. A new syndrome. Br Med J 1936;1:175–7.
3. Stahle J, Stahle C, Arenberg IK. Incidence of Menière's disease. Arch Otolaryngol 1978;104:99–102.
4. Häusler R, Toupet M, Guidetti G, et al. Menière's disease in children. Am J Otolaryngol 1987;8:187–93.
5. Pfaltz CR, Matéfi L. Menière's disease or syndrome? A critical review of diagnosis criteria. In: Vosteen KH, Schuknecht H, Pfaltz CR, et al, editors. Menière's disease: pathogenesis, diagnosis and treatment. Stuttgart (Germany): Thieme; 1981. p. 1–10.
6. Ballester M, Liard P, Vibert D, et al. Menière's disease in the elderly. Otol Neurotol 2002;23:73–8.
7. Da Costa SS, de Sousa LC, Piza MR. Meniere's disease: overview, epidemiology, and natural history. Otolaryngol Clin North Am 2002;35(3):455–95.
8. Mancini F, Catalani M, Carru M, et al. History of Meniere's disease and its clinical presentation. Otolaryngol Clin North Am 2002;35:565–80.
9. Katsarkas A. Hearing loss and vestibular dysfunction in Meniere's disease. Acta Otolaryngol 1996;116:185–8.
10. Meyerhoff WL, Paparella MM, Gudbrandsson FK. Clinical evaluation of Meniere's disease. Laryngoscope 1968;91:1663–8.
11. Oosterveld WJ. Meniere's disease, signs and symptoms. J Laryngol Otol 1980; 94:885–94.
12. Filipo R, Barbara M. Natural history of Meniere's disease: staging the patients or their symptoms? Acta Otolaryngol Suppl 1997;526:10–3.
13. Rodgers GK, Telischi FF. Meniere's disease in children. Otolaryngol Clin North Am 1997;30:1101–4.

14. Choung YH, Park K, Kim CH, et al. Rare cases of Menière's disease in children. J Laryngol Otol 2006;120:343–52.
15. Üneri A, Polat S. Vertigo, dizziness and imbalance in the elderly. J Laryngol Otol 2008;122:466–9.
16. Baloh RW, Jacobson K, Winder T. Drop attacks with Menière's syndrome. Ann Neurol 1990;28:384–7.
17. Merchant SN, Rauch SD, Nadol JB Jr. Menière's disease. Eur Arch Otorhinolaryngol 1995;252:63–75.
18. Black FO, Effron MZ, Burns DS. Diagnosis and management of drop attacks of vestibular origin: Tumarkin's otolithic crisis. Otolaryngol Head Neck Surg 1982; 90:256–62.
19. Kentala E, Havia M, Pyykkö I. Short-lasting drop attacks in Meniere's disease. Otolaryngol Head Neck Surg 2001;124(5):526–30.
20. Schuknecht H, Belal A. The utriculo-endolymphatic valve: its functional significance. J Laryngol Otol 1975;89:965–96.
21. House W. A theory of the production of symptoms of Meniere's disease. Otolaryngol Clin North Am 1968;1:375–88.
22. Ozeki H, Iwasaki S, Murofuschi T. Vestibular drop attack secondary to Meniere's disease results from unstable otolithic function. Acta Otolaryngol 2008;128: 887–91.
23. Merchant SN, Adams JC, Nadol JB. Pathophysiology of Ménière's syndrome: are symptoms caused by endolymphatic hydrops? Otol Neurotol 2005;26:74–81.
24. Ichimiya I, Adams JC, Kimura RS. Changes in immunostaining of cochleas with experimentally induced endolymphatic hydrops. Ann Otol Rhinol Laryngol 1994;103:457–68.
25. Nadol JB Jr, Adams JC, Kim JR. Degenerative changes in the organ of Corti and lateral cochlear wall in experimental endolymphatic hydrops and human Ménière's disease. Acta Otolaryngol Suppl 1995;519:47–59.
26. Shinomori Y, Kimura RS, Adams JC. Changes in immunostaining for Na+, K+ 2Cl-cotransporter 1, taurine and c-Jun N-terminal kinase in experimentally induced endolymphatic hydrops. ARO Abstr 2001;24:134.
27. Kikuchi T, Kimura RS, Paul DL, et al. Gap junctions in the rat cochlea: immunohistochemical and ultrastructural analysis. Anat Embryol 1995;191:101–18.
28. Steel KP. The benefits of recycling. Science 1999;285:1363–4.
29. Meyer zum Gottesberge AM, Kaufmann R. Is an imbalanced calcium homeostasis responsible for the experimentally induced endolymphatic hydrops? Acta Otolaryngol 1986;102:93–8.
30. Ninoyu O, Meyer zum Gottesberge AM. Changes in Ca++ activity and DC potential in experimentally induced endolymphatic hydrops. Arch Otorhinolaryngol 1986;243:106–7.
31. Salt AN, Inamura N, Thalmann R, et al. Calcium gradients in inner ear endolymph. Am J Otolaryngol 1989;10:371–5.
32. Anniko M. Development of otoconia. Am J Otolaryngol 1980;1:400–10.
33. Harada Y, Tagashira N. Metabolism of the otoconia. Biomed Res 1981;2(Suppl): 415–20.
34. Campos A, Crespo PV, Garcia JM, et al. The crystalline pattern of calcium in different topographical regions of the otoconial membrane. Acta Otolaryngol 1999;119:203–6.
35. Balsamo G, Avallone B, Del Genio F, et al. Calcification processes in the chick otoconia and calcium binding proteins: patterns of tetracycline incorporation and calbindin-D28K distribution. Hear Res 2000;148:1–8.

36. Lins U, Farina M, Kurc M, et al. The otoconia of the guinea pig utricle: internal structure, surface exposure, and interactions with the filament matrix. J Struct Biol 2000;131(1):67–78.
37. Vibert D, Kompis M, Häusler R. Benign paroxysmal positional vertigo in older women may be related to osteoporosis and osteopenia. Ann Otol Rhinol Laryngol 2003;112:885–9.
38. Vibert D, Sans A, Kompis M, et al. Ultrastructural changes in otoconia of osteoporotic rats. Audiol Neurootol 2008;13:293–301.
39. Harner SG, Kasperbauer JL, Facer GW, et al. Transtympanic gentamicin for Ménière's syndrome. Laryngoscope 1998;108:1446–9.
40. Lange G. 27 years' experience with transtympanic aminoglycoside treatment of Ménière's disease. Laryngorhinootologie 1995;74:720–3.
41. Ödkvist LM, Bergenius J, Moller C. When and how to use gentamicin in the treatment of Ménière's disease. Acta Otolaryngol Suppl 1997;526:54–7.
42. Montandon P, Guillemin P, Häusler R. Prevention of vertigo in Ménière's syndrome by means of transtympanic ventilation tubes. ORL J Otorhinolaryngol Relat Spec 1988;50:377–81.
43. Montandon P, Guillemin P, Häusler R. Treatment of Ménière's disease by means of minor surgical procedures: sacculotomy, cochleosacculotomy, transtympanic ventilation tubes. In: Nadol JB Jr, editor. Second International Symposium on Ménière's disease. Amsterdam: Kugler Publications; 1989. p. 503–8.
44. Thomsen J, Bonding P, Becker B, et al. The non-specific effect of endolymphatic sac surgery in treatment of Ménière's disease: a prospective, randomized controlled study comparing "classic" endolymphatic sac surgery with the insertion of a ventilating tube in the tympanic membrane. Acta Otolaryngol 1998;118:769–73.
45. Häusler R, Guillemin P, Montandon P. Surgical treatment of Ménière's disease by sacculotomy, cochlea-sacculotomy and transtympanic aerators. Rev Laryngol Otol Rhinol (Bord) 1991;112:149–52.
46. Ödkvist LM, Bergenius J. Drop attacks in Ménière's disease. Acta Otolaryngol Suppl 1988;455:82–5.
47. Langman AW, Linderman RC. Surgical labyrinthectomy in the older patient. Otolaryngol Head Neck Surg 1998;118:739–42.
48. Schwaber MK, Pensak ML, Reiber ME. Transmastoid labyrinthectomy in older patients. Laryngoscope 1995;105:1152–4.
49. Ishiyama G, Ishiyama A, Jacobson K, et al. Drop attacks in older patients secondary to an otologic cause. Neurology 2001;57:1103–6.

Allergy and Its Relation to Meniere's Disease

M. Jennifer Derebery, MD[a,b,*], Karen I. Berliner, PhD[a]

KEYWORDS

• Meniere's disease • Vertigo • Tinnitus • Hearing loss

In 1861, Prosper Ménière first associated dizziness with the inner ear.[1] Later, the syndrome of fluctuating sensorineural hearing loss, episodic vertigo, and tinnitus was named after him. Subsequently, the pathogenesis of Meniere's disease (MD) was found to be a hydropic distension of the endolymphatic system. In its guidelines for MD diagnosis and evaluation of treatment, the American Academy of Otolaryngology-Head and Neck Surgery (AAO-HNS) describes MD as a "clinical disorder defined as the idiopathic syndrome of endolymphatic hydrops... For clinical purposes (treatment and reporting), the presence of endolymphatic hydrops can be inferred during life by the presence of the syndrome of endolymphatic hydrops. This syndrome is defined as the presence of... recurrent, spontaneous, episodic vertigo; hearing loss; aural fullness; and tinnitus."[2] AAO-HNS guidelines further define the vertigo episodes as a "spontaneous rotational vertigo lasting at least 20 minutes." **Box 1** lists the classification of MD based on the AAO-HNS criteria.

The initial vertigo attack—the feeling of intense motion when sitting or standing still—can cause the subject to fall to the ground and is accompanied by nausea and vomiting. An incidence of 15 per 100,000 and a prevalence of 218 per 100,000 have been reported for MD in the United States.[4] Although idiopathic, MD has been ascribed to various causes, including trauma, viral infections, metabolic disorders, allergies, and autoimmune factors. The first author emphasizes that MD, at the time of writing, is idiopathic. She believes that there may be some genetic predisposition to the development of MD and/or endolymphatic hydrops, with the final "insult" resulting in disease development being inflammatory or a dysregulation of ion channels. She does not believe that MD, per se, is caused by allergies; rather, in some patients who probably have a genetic predisposition, an allergic reaction produced by a food and/or inhalant allergen may stimulate an inflammatory reaction resulting in the development of symptoms. In this article, the authors specifically look at the evidence, historical and

[a] Clinical Studies Department, House Ear Institute, 2100 West Third Street, 5th Floor, Los Angeles, CA 90057, USA
[b] Department of Otolaryngology, USC Keck School of Medicine, Los Angeles, CA, USA
* Corresponding author. Clinical Studies Department, House Ear Institute, 2100 West Third Street, 5th Floor, Los Angeles, CA 90057.
E-mail address: jderebery@hei.org

Otolaryngol Clin N Am 43 (2010) 1047–1058
doi:10.1016/j.otc.2010.05.004
0030-6665/10/$ – see front matter © 2010 Elsevier Inc. All rights reserved.

oto.theclinics.com

Box 1
Classification of Meniere's Disease based on the AAO-HNS criteria

Certain Meniere's Disease

- Definite MD plus histopathologic confirmation

Definite Meniere's Disease

- Two or more definite spontaneous episodes of rotational vertigo for 20 minutes or longer
- Audiometrically documented hearing loss (uni- or bilateral) on at least one occasion
- Tinnitus or aural fullness in the affected ear
- Other causes excluded, such as vestibular schwannoma

Probable Meniere's Disease

- One definite episode of rotational vertigo
- Audiometrically documented hearing loss (uni- or bilateral) on at least one occasion
- Tinnitus or aural fullness in the affected ear
- Other causes excluded

Possible Meniere's Disease

- Episodic vertigo of the Meniere's type without documented hearing loss, or
- Sensorineural hearing loss (uni- or bilateral, fluctuating or fixed, with dysequilibrium but without definite episodes of vertigo
- Other causes excluded[3]

---

current, linking some cases of MD to an underlying allergic state and do not address other potential stimuli, such as viral antigen or autoimmune reaction other than the Type I Gell and Coombs reaction characterized by allergy.

In this article, the authors review the immunology of the inner ear followed by literature from 2002 to 2009 on MD, allergy, and autoimmunity.

REVIEW OF IMMUNOLOGY

The inner ear has little exposure to pathogens and few resident cells that are associated with immunologic function. In the past, this led to assumptions that it was immunologically privileged, similar to the brain. More recent research indicates that the inner ear is actually more immunoresponsive than the brain.[5] The labyrinth exhibits a blood-labyrinthine barrier analogous to the blood-brain barrier, which maintains the cochlea's unique ionic characteristics. There is no lymphatic drainage from the inner ear, and, although immunoglobulins are present in the perilymph, the amount is only one-thousandth of that in the serum.[6]

The inner ear demonstrates cellular and humoral immunity. Most leukocytes enter the cochlea via the spiral modiolar vein.[7] The innate immunity of the cochlea has been suggested to allow an adaptive local response to antigen challenge.[8] Hashimoto and colleagues[8] have suggested that the inner ear may be primed by lipopolysaccharides or other viral or bacterial antigens, resulting in the upregulation of interleukin (IL)-1C in the spiral ligament fibrocytes permitting leukocytes to enter. Subsequently, in those having lymphocytes primed to react against inner-ear antigens, an initiated immune response may result in local inflammation. Altermatt and colleagues[9] have suggested that the seat of immunoactivity in the inner ear seems to be the endolymphatic sac

(ES) and duct. Immunoglobulin (Ig) G, IgM, IgA, and secretory component are found in the ES, and numerous plasma cells and macrophages reside in the perisaccular connective tissue.

Additionally, the labyrinth exhibits active components of allergic reactivity. Mast cells have been identified in the perisaccular connective tissue. Following sensitization, IgE-mediated degranulation of mast cells has resulted in eosinophilic infiltration of the perisaccular connective tissue, and, clinically, the production of endolymphatic hydrops.[10]

The ES is capable of processing antigen and producing its own local antibody response.[11,12] Surgical destruction of the ES results in decreased antigen and antibody responses.[12] The highly vascular subepithelial space of the ES contains numerous fenestrated blood vessels,[13] with arterial branches of the posterior meningeal artery supplying the ES and duct.[14] Although the labyrinth is protected by the blood-labyrinthine barrier, the posterior meningeal artery is fenestrated, offering a peripheral portal of circulation. Fenestrated vessels supplying organs involved in absorption (eg, kidney, choroid) are especially susceptible to damage by immune complex deposition.

Despite evidence of immune activity, only 30% of patients with MD show a true autoantibody response on Western blot assay to specific anticochlear antibody.[15] Tests of abnormal cell-mediated immunity are either inconsistent or normal, even in patients with known causes of inner ear autoimmune dysfunction, including Cogan syndrome.[15] Despite increased understanding of labyrinthine immunoreactivity, a reliable laboratory marker has not been developed to prove autoimmune or allergic causation in patients with suspected inflammatory hearing loss.

POSSIBLE MECHANISMS INVOLVING ALLERGY

The first published report that MD was believed to be provoked by an allergic reaction was in 1923.[16] Inhalant and food allergies have been linked with MD symptoms.[17] Many of MD's clinical characteristics suggest an underlying inflammatory, if not autoimmune, cause, such as its propensity to wax and wane with periods of remission. It is also bilateral in a significant number of cases.[18,19]

There are different possible mechanisms by which an allergic reaction produces MD symptoms.[20] First, the ES itself could be a target organ of the allergic reaction. The sac's peripheral and fenestrated blood vessels could allow antigen entry, stimulating mast cell degranulation in the perisaccular connective tissue. The resulting inflammatory mediator release could affect the sac's filtering capability, resulting in a toxic accumulation of metabolic products and interfering with hair cell function. Also, the fenestrated blood vessels to the ES could be pharmacologically vulnerable to the effects of vasoactive mediators such as histamine, which are released in a distal allergic reaction. The unique blood supply of the interosseus ES would serve as a portal for these mediators to exert a direct pharmacologic effect. The potent vasodilating effects of histamine or other mediators could affect the resorptive capacity of the ES. Yan and colleagues[21] have shown that Waldeyer ring in the nasopharynx is the anatomic site of T-cell homing to the ES. In systemically sensitized rodents, intranasal antigen stimulation with keyhole limpet hemocyanin in Waldeyer ring resulted in an antigen-specific reaction in the ES and perilymphatic vessels, suggesting that viral or allergic antigen could be processed in the nasopharynx with the resulting specific immune reaction occurring at the ES.

A second possible mechanism involves the production of a circulating immune complex, such as a food antigen, which is then deposited through the fenestrated blood vessels of the ES, producing inflammation. An increased incidence of circulating immune complexes in the serum has been described in MD and allergic rhinitis.[22,23] The inflammatory response resulting from the deposition of immune complexes along vascular basement membranes is the hallmark of an immune complex disease. Although the binding of the complexes to the cell membranes facilitates their phago-cytosis, it also results in the release of tissue-damaging enzymes. This is believed to be the mechanism of unexplained sensorineural hearing loss in patients with Wegener granulomatosis, a prototype immune-complex–mediated disease. On examining the temporal bones of patients with Wegener granulomatosis and unexplained sensori-neural hearing loss, the cochlea is found to be normal; the pathology occurs in the ES.[24]

Alternatively, circulating immune complexes may be deposited in the stria, causing the normally intact blood-labyrinthine barrier to leak as a result of increased vascular permeability. In addition to disrupting normal ionic and fluid balance in the extracapil-lary spaces, this could facilitate the entry of autoantibodies into the inner ear.

A third possible mechanism is a viral antigen-allergic interaction. A predisposing viral upper respiratory infection in childhood (eg, mumps, herpes) antigenically stimulates Waldeyer ring, with subsequent T-cell homing to the ES,[21] resulting in a chronic low-grade inflammation. This is not enough initially to result in hearing loss or vertigo, but it does produce mild impairment of ES absorption. Later in adult life, something in the system stimulates excess fluid production. Several investigators have assumed that viral infections play a direct or indirect role in the cause of MD. Viruses are also capable of exacerbating allergic symptoms by several mechanisms. Live and ultraviolet light-inactivated viruses have been shown to enhance histamine release, an effect believed to be mediated by interferon. Viruses can also damage epithelial surfaces, thereby enhancing antigen entry and increasing the responsiveness of target organs to hista-mine. It has long been noted that patients with poorly controlled allergy are more likely than nonallergic persons to develop upper and lower respiratory viral infections.

EPIDEMIOLOGY

In a survey the authors performed of 734 patients with MD, the prevalence of skin test-confirmed concurrent allergic disease was 41%.[25] Although the prevalence of allergic rhinitis is often quoted as 20% or more, the recent Allergies in America report, the largest survey to date regarding prevalence and disease burden of allergic rhinitis, found that physician-diagnosed allergic rhinitis in patients with rhinitic symptoms is 14%.[26] Hence, the prevalence of physician-diagnosed allergy in American patients diagnosed with MD is almost 3 times that of the general population.[25] In a more recent survey of patients with MD, the authors found that patients reported a 58% rate of allergy history, and again, a 41% rate of positive skin or in vitro test.[19]

In his original description, Prosper Ménière suggested an association between migraine and MD.[1] Many authors have subsequently noted paroxysmal headache inde-pendently occurring in many patients with MD.[27–29] Radtke and colleagues[30] published a well-designed prospective trial based on strict diagnostic criteria, which established an increased lifetime prevalence of migraine in patients diagnosed with MD.

A recent study reported an increased incidence of self-reported migraine and allergic rhinitis in patients with MD, as compared with a control group of age- and sex-matched patients without MD attending an otolaryngology clinic.[31] Sen and colleagues[31] used a Web-based questionnaire to recruit 108 patients with MD and a control group of 100 patients attending the otolaryngology clinic for other prob-lems. The migraine prevalence in MD sufferers was 39% compared with 18% in the control group, whereas the prevalence of allergy in those with MD was 51.9% compared with 23% in the control group. In the MD group, a history of allergy was significantly more prevalent in patients with migraine (71%) than in those without migraine (39%). There was no such link between allergy and migraine in the control group, with the combination of allergy and migraine 9 times more prevalent in the MD group (adds ratio 9.23; 95% confidence interval 3.11–27.32).

The study by Sen and colleagues[31] is interesting because it suggests that in that large subset of patients with MD who also have migraine, the vast majority report an additional diagnosis of allergy. One weakness of their Web-based questionnaire is that the allergy history is obtained by asking subjects whether they or their family members suffer from any allergy, without confirmatory skin or in vitro testing. However, all patients—control and MD groups—were asked the same question and gave such differing responses as to add credence to the supposition that there is a much higher incidence of allergy and migraine in patients with M.D.

More recently, Ibekwe and colleagues[32] reported that 32% of patients presenting to a clinic in Nigeria and diagnosed by an otolaryngologist with MD also had associated features of migraine, compared with 5.3% of the overall population. Migraine without aura ("common migraine") was the most common presentation, occurring in approximately 62.5% of patients. This study shows that a history of allergy is much more common in patients with MD and migraine than in those without migraine. The investigators suggest that the vasodilatory effects of allergy or possible extravasations of immune complexes may serve as a common pathway for migraine and MD.Although a weakness of this paper is the small number of patients reported, there is a striking similarity in the prevalence of migraine in this study and that reported by Sen.

Although the list of causes for migraine is extensive, it has long been noted that allergic reactions were a common trigger in many sufferers. There are striking similarities in symptom presentation and vascular changes between MD, allergy, and migraines. All 3 tend to recur cyclically, and sufferers are often able to note a cause and effect between a particular suspected "exposure" or event and the subsequent development of symptoms. All the entities also show similar vascular changes during the course of symptom production: vasoconstriction, vasodilatation, and plasma extravasations. There is an elevation in IgG-containing immune complexes in the meningeal vessels of patients with migraine and in the subepithelial layer of the ES in patients with MD.[32] The elevated level of circulating immune complexes in MD has already been mentioned.[23]

Ibekwe hypothesized that there may be a common defective ion channel in both disease states, with the predominant expression in the inner ear and brain, resulting in a local increase in extracellular potassium and the production of symptoms.

PATHOPHYSIOLOGY

Paparella and Djalilian[33] provide an excellent article for the practitioner of the temporal bone correlates of the clinical symptoms of MD. They review various theorized causes of MD symptoms including allergy. They conclude that the fundamental cause of MD is probably a multifactorial inheritance, suggesting that the most likely predisposing factors are hypoplasia of the mastoid air cell system, vestibular aqueduct, and ES and the other physical abnormalities that have been frequently reported in patients with MD.

The authors also believe that MD is probably multifactorial in cause. It is not their contention that MD is caused by allergy. However, if they accept that most patients with MD do have an anatomic abnormality including a smaller than average ES size, factors that may affect either excessive endolymph production or reduction of endolymph absorption may promote MD symptoms. Inflammatory stimulation by an inhaled or ingested allergen in a genetically predisposed individual should be considered as one possible trigger.

IMMUNOPATHOLOGY

Savastano and colleagues[34] studied the validity of serologic nonspecific immune tests in determining a possible role of immunopathology in a series of 200 patients with MD compared with a control group of 50 healthy blood donors. All patients and controls had no known diagnosis of autoimmune disease or steroid treatment. Results indicated negative or insignificant levels of IgG, IgM, IgA, erythrocyte sedimentation rate, C-reactive protein, complement factors, and cryoglobulins in most patients. However, more than half had significant elevations in levels of circulating immune complexes. Rates of elevation of circulating immune complexes, lymphocyte subpopulations (especially IL-2 receptor), and autoantibodies were higher in the MD group than in controls.

Savastano and colleagues[34] also attempted to relate immunologic findings to disease severity, using the 1985 AAO-HNS Pearson and Brackmann classification of disability for reporting results in MD treatment (it is unclear why they did not use the currently accepted AAO-HNS functional disability scale from the 1995 guidelines). In the 1985 system, grade I exhibits mild or no disability, with intermittent or continuous dizziness precluding work in a hazardous environment; grade II, moderate disability with intermittent or continuous dizziness/unsteadiness requiring employment in a sedentary occupation; and grade III, severe disability/disabling symptoms precluding gainful employment. There was a significant relationship between disease severity and test abnormalities for circulating immune complexes, CD4, and CD4-to-CD8 ratio, with the highest rate of serologic abnormalities found in group III with disabling symptoms and the lowest rate, in group I. A trend was also found for differences in C-reactive protein, C3 complement, and early T-activation.

Elevated circulating immune complexes in patients with MD have been reported by Brookes[22] and by Derebery and colleagues.[23] It would have been interesting for Savastano and colleagues[34] to have done a subanalysis of patients with bilateral MD (not identified in the text). Derebery and colleagues[23] have found a direct relationship between larger elevations in circulating immune complexes and disease bilaterality.

The study by Savastano and colleagues[34] adds credence to a possible underlying inflammatory cause in most patients with MD. The investigators suggest that monitoring serum levels of circulating immune complexes, CD4, and CD4-to-CD8 ratios may be useful as prognostic markers of disease progression. However, they did not elaborate on possible treatments, immune-suppressive or allergic, resulting from their conclusions.

Keles and colleagues[35] performed another study of MD immunopathology; they attempted to evaluate the possible role of allergy in producing MD symptoms by examining the cytokine profiles, allergic parameters, and lymphocyte subgroups of patients with MD versus controls.

Forty-six adult patients with classic MD were compared with an identical number of healthy volunteers in the same age group and socioeconomic class living in the same region of Turkey. These researchers performed an extensive immune profile, measuring monoclonal CD4, CD8, CD23 antibodies, interferon (IFN)-H, IL-4, total serum IgE, and antigen-specific IgE pertaining to regionally important tree pollens, molds, and common foods in the local diet.

Significant differences were found between the patients with MD and the controls in CD4, CD4/CD8, CD23, IFN-H, and IL-4 levels. Keles and colleagues[35] also found significant positive correlations between levels of CD23 and total serum IgE, CD8 and total serum IgE, CD4/CD8 and IgE, and CD23 and CD8, although correlation coefficients were not provided for the reader to determine strength of the relationships. Elevation of total serum IgE was found in 43.3% of the MD group compared with only 19.5% of the control group. Additionally, 67.3% of the patients with MD gave a positive history of allergy, whereas the same was found in only 34.7% of the control group. Significant elevations of antigen-specific IgE in the patients with MD were not present in the control group.

Keles and colleagues[35] suggest that future therapies could potentially be beneficial, such as suppressing production of IL-4 and IL-1 or stimulating a helper T1 (T_H1) cell predominance by the application of BCG vaccine. This study does not change the current treatment parameters for MD. However, it documents that unselected patients with MD have serologic findings that correlate strongly with atopy.

TREATMENT

The authors review several studies related to treatment of MD on immunologic aspects of the disease. Jeck-Thole and Wagner[36] published a review of safety data on betahistine, which is often sold under the trade name Serc (Solvay Pharmaceuticals, Marietta, GA, USA). Betahistine contains a structural analogue of histamine and is prescribed in the treatment of vestibular disorders such as MD for symptomatic treatment of vertigo. Betahistine is said to be the most commonly prescribed medication for MD. Although not currently available in the United States, it can be obtained by compounding pharmacies or through sources in Canada or Europe. The typical adult dose is 16 mg thrice daily. The reader occasionally may see a patient with MD using betahistine and reporting good clinical results.

In the United States, the most commonly prescribed medications for treating symptoms of MD are antihistamines (eg, meclizine, diphenhydramine, dimenhydrinate). Therefore, it might appear to be counterintuitive to prescribe a histamine analogue to treat these same symptoms. In tissue, histamine is primarily stored in mast cells and may be released by various drugs, venoms, or allergens, resulting in hypersensitivity reactions, gastric acid secretion, and increased capillary permeability. In association with the peripheral actions of histamine, its function as a central neurotransmitter was postulated. Subsequently, various receptor subtypes were described, including histamine H_1, H_2, H_3 and, eventually, H_4.[37,38]

Betahistine acts as a neurotransmitter modulator of the complex histaminergic receptor system with no known affinity for any other receptors.[39] Betahistine is a weak partial H_1-receptor agonist with a distinctly lower affinity than histamine. It has almost no affinity for the H_2 receptor, having extremely weak effects on gastric secretion.[40] In contrast, betahistine shows a potent antagonistic effect on the H_3 receptor. The H_3 heteroreceptor, belonging to a class of presynaptic receptors, is involved in the synthesis and release of histamine and other neurotransmitters, including dopamine, γ-aminobutyric acid, acetylcholine, norepinephrine, and serotonin.[41] Actions that are mediated by the H_1 receptor are blocked by negative H_3-receptor feedback. Betahistine has an antagonistic effect on the H_3 receptor followed by an increased histamine release. Betahistine's H_3-receptor antagonistic action is believed to be responsible for improvement in the inner ear microcirculation and subsequent reduction of endolymphatic pressure.[42,43] Betahistine has also been shown to inhibit the basal spike generation of the vestibular neurons in the lateral and medial vestibular nuclei, both crucial for controlling posture. A recent meta-analysis of treatment with betahistine in treating vertigo in non-MD patients has shown it to be efficacious.[44]

In terms of side effects or drug interaction, betahistine is nonsedating and free from psychomotor impairment. Theoretically, because betahistine and histamine are similar, betahistine could interact with an antihistaminic agent, such as diphenhydramine or cetirizine, or even induce or support hypersensitivity reactions with regard to the H_1-agonistic quality. However, betahistine affinity at the receptor site has been shown to be significantly weaker than histamine affinity. Betahistine-induced histamine release from mast cells has also not been described.[45]

INDICATIONS FOR TESTING

Classically, Powers described suggestive history including a seasonal relationship of symptoms (eg, hearing loss, vertigo attacks) and the presence of other symptoms suggesting allergy, such as rhinitis, as indicators.[17] These are actually a useful guide. The first author feels that other details of history are useful guides, including bilateral symptoms, strong family history of allergy, a history of childhood allergy that one has outgrown, and obvious factors such as the production of MD symptoms within a short time after exposure to a food or inhaled antigen.

There are varying thoughts on the relative sensitivity versus specificity of various tests, including intradermal, intradermal titration, intradermal dilutional provocative food testing, and in vitro. Readers are encouraged to perform their own review of the subject. The authors would suggest that irrespective of testing type, the patient be tested with inhalant and food antigens, despite the acknowledged lesser sensitivity of food testing when compared with inhalant.

Their preferred method of testing is intradermal titration, or, less so, prick testing, with single dilution intradermal testing in the case of negative results with a prick test. They have observed that the reactivity of patients with suspected inhalant allergic triggers to their MD symptoms is often relatively low, typically in the range of 1/500 weight/volume of antigen.[46] Likewise, Topuz and colleagues[47] also noted that there was a large increase of abnormal electrocochleographic (ECOG) results from pre-prick testing to post-testing in patients with MD (29% of diseased ears vs 78% post-testing) and that the inner ear did not appear to require a strong antigen dose to be objectively stimulated. Similar ECOG changes have also been noted in patients with MD who have been tested with dietary antigen stimulation by provocative food testing, nasal provocation with inhalant antigens, and prick testing.[48] The purpose of testing for allergy is to establish objectively whether a patient is allergic to a particular allergen rather than to infer that the amount of antigen that produces a positive skin test directly relates to the type or severity of induced symptoms.

TREATMENT OUTCOME STUDIES

The authors used a questionnaire on symptoms to evaluate the effect of specific allergy immunotherapy and food elimination of suspected food allergens on patients with MD for whom allergy treatment had been recommended.[20] The 113 patients treated by desensitization and diet showed a significant improvement in allergy and MD symptoms after treatment. The patient ratings of frequency, severity, and interference with daily activities of their MD symptoms also seemed better after allergy treatment compared with ratings from the control group of 24 untreated patients. Results indicated that patients with MD can show improvement in tinnitus and vertigo symptoms when receiving specific allergy therapy, suggesting that the inner ear may also be a direct or indirect target of an allergic reaction.

Because the study asked patients to retrospectively rate their pretreatment symptoms, a prospective study was undertaken in which 68 patients completed the questionnaire before and at an average of 23 months after treatment.[49] Severity of vertigo, tinnitus, and unsteadiness decreased significantly, as did frequency of vertigo, frequency and interference of unsteadiness, and ratings on the AAO-HNS disability scale. Quality of life improved significantly on 4 of 8 Medical Outcomes Study 36-Item Short Form Health Survey (SF-36) scales. Initial SF-36 scores indicated that patients with MD and allergy have poorer scores than the general US adult population on several quality-of-life aspects. Paired comparisons between SF-36 scale scores at initial and follow-up intervals identified significant improvements in subtests that were less than normal initially. Statistical analyses strongly suggested that these improvements were independent of natural history and of other medical treatment for MD that the patients may have received during the immunotherapy period.

A weakness of these and other studies is that there are no control groups receiving saline injections or given diets eliminating foods that were negative on testing. The authors have observed that patients with MD are reluctant to commit to months or a year of possible placebo injections to prove that immunotherapy may help improve symptoms of vertigo, hearing loss, and/or tinnitus. Presently, they rely on using statistical control and research that demonstrates the ability of allergy immunotherapy to down-regulate T_H2 cell–driven inflammatory responses in patients with allergic rhinitis and asthma.[50] If MD is believed to be a chronic condition with an inflammatory component, it is logical that down-regulating the production and release of proinflammatory and vasoactive mediators promoting fluid extravasation and/or retention could help lessen symptoms. This is the rationale for using steroids and restricting dietary salt in patients with MD.

The classic first-generation antihistamines commonly used for their desired anticholinergic effects to lessen vertigo severity do not change the underlying pathology of hydropic distention of the endolymphatic space. Pharmacologically, these agents have limited effect and do not block the effects of other inflammatory mediators, such as leukotrienes, released with mast cell degranulation. In the authors' experience, nonsedating antihistamines have limited benefit in treating vertigo and/or dizziness. Effective immunotherapy with its induced immunologic changes can prevent mast cell degranulation. Additionally, an appropriate elimination diet for documented food allergies can prevent an immune-mediated reaction.

In the authors' clinical experience, the symptoms of MD are generally better controlled, with fewer vertigo attacks and more stable hearing, in those patients with allergy and MD whose underlying allergic disorder is down-regulated with immunotherapy and/or dietary avoidance of reactive food allergens. The ideal proof of the role of allergy in a large subset of patients who develop MD would be a double-blind, placebo-controlled trial of immunotherapy for the minimum of 2 years, as required by the AAO-HNS for evaluating the effects of surgical procedures for MD; however, realistically, recruiting patients for such a study would be a challenge because of the potentially disabling symptoms of MD.

SUMMARY

The prevalence of migraine and atopy is much higher in patients with MD than in the normal population. Unselected patients with MD have serologic findings that correlate with underlying atopy and inflammation. Indications for allergy testing in a patient with MD should include a seasonal or food relationship to symptom production, a known history of allergy or clear allergic symptoms in a patient with MD, and a known past childhood history or a strong family history of allergy. Additional consideration should be given for testing in those patients with bilateral MD. Although there are no double-blind, placebo-controlled trials comparing outcomes of patients with MD treated with specific allergy immunotherapy, clinical case reports strongly suggest that such treatment lessens severity and frequency of vertigo and results in more stable hearing. Objective outcomes of successful medical and surgical treatment of MD symptoms have been established and published and may be used as a reference for assessing treatment response by specific allergy immunotherapy or dietary elimination of food allergy.

REFERENCES

1. Ménière P. Pathologieauriculaire: mémoire sur des lésions de l'oreille interne donnant lieu a des symtomes de congestion cerebrale apoplectiforme. Gaz Med (Paris) 1861;16:597–601.
2. American Academy of Otolaryngology—Head and Neck Foundation. Committee on hearing and equilibrium guidelines for the diagnosis and evaluation of therapy in Ménière's disease. Otolaryngol Head Neck Surg 1995;113:181–5.
3. Hamid MA. Ménière's disease. Pract Neurol 2009;9:157–62.
4. Wladislavosky-Waserman P, Facer GW, Mokri B, et al. Ménière's disease: a 30-year epidemiologic and clinical study in Rochester, MN, 1951–1980. Laryngoscope 1984;94:1098–102.
5. Harris JP, Keithley EM, Ballenger S. Autoimmune inner ear disease. In: Snow JB, Ballenger JJ, editors. Otorhinolaryngology head and neck surgery. 16th edition. Hamilton (Canada): BC Decker; 2003. p. 396–407.
6. Harris JP. Immunology of the inner ear: response of the inner ear to antigen challenge. Otolaryngol Head Neck Surg 1983;91:18–23.
7. Stearns GS, Keithley EM, Harris JP. Development of high endothelial venule-like characteristics in the spiral modiolar vein induced by viral labyrinthitis. Laryngoscope 1993;103:890–8.
8. Hashimoto S, Billings P, Harris JP, et al. Innate immunity contributes to cochlear adaptive immune responses. Audiol Neurootol 2005;10:35–43.
9. Altermatt HJ, Gebbers JO, Müller C, et al. Human endolymphatic sac: evidence for a role in inner ear immune defence. ORL J Otorhinolaryngol Relat Spec 1990; 52:143–8.
10. Uno K, Miyamura K, Kanzaki Y, et al. Type I allergy in the inner ear of the guinea pig. Ann Otol Rhinol Laryngol 1992;101(Suppl 157):78–81.
11. Harris JP. Immunology of the inner ear: evidence of local antibody production. Ann Otol Rhinol Laryngol 1984;93:157–62.
12. Tomiyama S, Harris JP. The role of the endolymphatic sac in inner ear immunity. Acta Otolaryngol 1987;103:182–8.
13. Wackym PA, Friberg U, Linthicum FH Jr, et al. Human endolymphatic sac: morphologic evidence of immunologic function. Ann Otol Rhinol Laryngol 1987; 96:276–81.
14. Gadre AK, Fayad JN, O'Leary MJ, et al. Arterial supply of the human endolymphatic duct and sac. Otolaryngol Head Neck Surg 1993;108:141–8.
15. Harris JP, Ryan AF. Fundamental immune mechanisms of the brain and inner ear. Otolaryngol Head Neck Surg 1995;112:639–53.

16. Duke W. Ménière's syndrome caused by allergy. JAMA 1923;81:2179–82.
17. Powers WH. Allergic factors in Ménière's disease. Trans Am Acad Ophthalmol Otolaryngol 1973;77:22.
18. House JW, Doherty JK, Fisher LM, et al. Ménière's disease: prevalence of contralateral ear involvement. Otol Neurotol 2006;27:355–61.
19. Derebery MJ, Berliner KI. Characteristics, onset and progression in Ménière's disease. In: Lim DJ, editor. Proceedings of the 5th International Symposium on Ménière's disease and inner ear homeostasis disorders. Los Angeles (CA): House Ear Institute; 2005. p. 128–30.
20. Derebery MJ. Allergic management of Ménière's disease: an outcome study. Otolaryngol Head Neck Surg 2000;122:174–82.
21. Yan Z, Wang JB, Gong SS, et al. Cell proliferation in the endolymphatic sac in situ after the rat Waldeyer ring equivalent immunostimulation. Laryngoscope 2003; 113:1609–14.
22. Brookes GB. Circulating immune complexes in Ménière's disease. Arch Otolaryngol Head Neck Surg 1986;112:536–40.
23. Derebery MJ, Rao VS, Siglock TJ, et al. Ménière's disease: an immune complex-mediated illness? Laryngoscope 1991;101:225–9.
24. Leone CA, Feghali JG, Linthicum FH Jr. Endolymphatic sac: possible role in autoimmune sensorineural hearing loss. Ann Otol Rhinol Laryngol 1984;93: 208–9.
25. Derebery MJ, Berliner KI. Prevalence of allergy in Ménière's disease. Otolaryngol Head Neck Surg 2000;123:69–75.
26. Allergies in America. A landmark survey of nasal allergy sufferers. Available at: http://www.myallergiesinamerica.com/. Accessed November 20, 2009.
27. Atkinson M. Migraine and Ménière's disease. Arch Otolaryngol 1962;75:48–51.
28. Hinchcliffe R. Headache and Ménière's disease. Acta Otolaryngol 1967;63: 384–90.
29. Dolowitz DA. Ménière's—an inner ear seizure. Laryngoscope 1979;89:67–77.
30. Radtke A, Lempert T, Gresty MA, et al. Migraine and Ménière's disease: is there a link? Neurology 2002;5:1700–4.
31. Sen P, Georgalas C, Papesch M. Co-morbidity of migraine and Ménière's disease: is allergy the link? J Laryngol Otol 2005;119:455–60.
32. Ibekwe TS, Fasunla JA, Ibekwe PU, et al. Migraine and Ménière's disease: two different phenomena with frequently observed concomitant occurrences. J Natl Med Assoc 2008;100:334–8.
33. Paparella MM, Djalilian HR. Etiology, pathophysiology of symptoms, and pathogenesis of Ménière's disease. Otolaryngol Clin North Am 2002;35: 529–45.
34. Savastano M, Giacomelli L, Marioni G. Non-specific immunological determinations in Ménière's disease: any role in clinical practice? Eur Arch Otorhinolaryngol 2007;264:15–9.
35. Keles E, Godekmerdan A, Kalidag T, et al. Ménière's disease and allergy: allergens and cytokines. J Laryngol Otol 2004;118:688–93.
36. Jeck-Thole S, Wagner W. Betahistine: a retrospective synopsis of safety data. Drug Saf 2006;29:1049–59.
37. Hill SJ, Ganellin CR, Timmerman H, et al. International Union of Pharmacology, XIII. Classification of histamine receptors. Pharmacol Rev 1997;49:253–77.
38. Liu C, Ma XJ, Jiang X, et al. Cloning and pharmacological characterization of a fourth histamine receptor (H_4) expressed in bone marrow. Mol Pharmacol 2001;5:420–6.

39. Arrang JM, Garbarg M, Quach TT, et al. Actions of betahistine at histamine receptors in the brain. Eur J Pharmacol 1985;111:73–84.

40. Curwain BP, Holton P, Spencer J. The effect of betahistine on gastric acid secretion and mucosal blood flow in conscious dogs. Br J Pharmacol 1972;46:351–4.

41. West RE, Zweig A, Shih NY, et al. Identification of two H3-histamine receptors subtypes. Mol Pharmacol 1990;38:610–3.

42. Laurikainen EL, Miller JM, Nutall AL. The vascular mechanism of action betahistine in the inner ear of the guinea pig. Eur Arch Otorhinolaryngol 1998;255: 119–23.

43. Dziadziola JK, Laurikian EL, Rachel JD. Betahistine increases vestibular blood flow. Otolaryngol Head Neck Surg 1999;120:400–5.

44. Della PC, Guidetti G, Eandi M. Betahistine in the treatment of vertiginous syndromes: a meta-analysis. Acta Otorhinolaryngol Ital 2006;26:208–15.

45. Kohno S, Nakao S, Ogawa K, et al. Possible participation of histamine H3-receptors in the regulation of anaphylactic histamine release from isolated rat peritoneal mast cells. Jpn J Pharmacol 1994;66:173–80.

46. Derebery MJ, Valenzuela S, et al. Ménière's syndrome and allergy. Otolaryngol Clin North Am 1992;25(1):213–24.

47. Topuz B, Ogmen G, Ardiç FN, et al. Provocation of endolymphatic hydrops with a Prick test in Menieres disease. Adv Ther 2007;24(4):819–25.

48. Gibbs SR, Mabry RL, Roland PS, et al. ECOG changes after intranasal allergen challenge: a possible diagnostic tool in patients with Ménière's disease. Otolaryngol Head Neck Surg 1999;121:283–4.

49. Derebery MJ, Berliner KI. Allergic management in Ménière's disease: a prospective study. Presented at the American Academy of Otolaryngic Allergy Annual Meeting. Orlando (FL), September 19, 2003.

50. Yang X. Does allergen immunotherapy alter the natural course of allergic disorders? Drugs 2001;61:365–74.

Magnetic Resonance Imaging of the Inner Ear in Meniere's Disease

Ilmari Pyykkö, MD[a],*, Jing Zou, MD[a], Dennis Poe, MD[a,b], Tsutomu Nakashima, MD[c], Shinji Naganawa, MD[d]

KEYWORDS

- MRI • Meniere's disease • Membrane leakage
- Stria vascularis porocity • Round-window administration

Magnetic resonance imaging (MRI) of the delicate structures of the inner ear has been addressed with the use of high field strength magnets and various contrast agents in recent years.[1,2] The inner ear is housed in dense bone and subdivided into different fluid-filled compartments that make imaging challenging. Methodological development in imaging techniques that has allowed separation of bone from fluid and contrast agent and increase of the magnetic field strength has improved spectral resolution, signal-to-noise and contrast-to-noise ratios and reduced scan acquisition times.[3,4] These properties are particularly helpful in the attempt to resolve details between the minute fluid-filled spaces within the cochlea. Contrast agents to enhance or darken fluid or tissue signal help to visualize regions of interest and efforts are now being made to create biologic tags using these agents for molecular imaging at the level of cellular processes.

Visualization of endolymphatic hydrops (EH) in Meniere's disease has always been an important goal for clinicians, but hitherto has been limited to postmortem histology. Histologic quantification of hydrops has been accomplished using a 3-step grading system to record the position of the Reissner's membrane. Scientific reports have

This study was supported by the EU on integrated project Nanoear (NMP4-CT-2006-026556) and by research grants from the Ministry of Health, Labor & Welfare, and the Ministry of Education, Culture, Sports, Science & Technology in Japan.

[a] Department of Otolaryngology, University of Tampere, Teiskontie 35, 33520, Tampere, Finland

[b] Department of Otology & Laryngology, Harvard Medical School, Boston, MA, USA

[c] Department of Otolaryngology, Nagoya University School of Medicine, 65, Tsurumai-cho, Showa-ku, Nagoya, Japan

[d] Department of Radiology, Nagoya University School of Medicine, 65, Tsurumai-cho, Showa-ku, Nagoya, Japan

* Corresponding author.

E-mail address: Ilmari.pyykko@pshp.fi

doi:10.1016/j.otc.2010.06.001
oto.theclinics.com

not yet been capable of systematically quantifying the extent of vestibular hydrops in vivo and establishing a correlation with symptoms, degree of hearing loss, and cochlear fluid dynamics. These difficulties are probably due in part to the variation in symptoms over time, including fluctuations in hearing level. This loose time dependency of symptoms is reflected in the grading of Meniere's disease based on the American Academy of Otolaryngology-Head and Neck Surgery (AAO-HNS) classification scale.[5] Requirements of AAO-HNS leave the distinction of certain elements of Meniere's disease for histologic evaluation made by post mortem. In addition, other diseases that may be related to EH are not officially recognized, although in many instances the fluctuant hearing loss and recurrent attacks of rotatory vertigo occur, such as subtypes of sudden deafness and autoimmune disorders.

MRI diagnosis of Meniere's disease was challenging until recent years. In humans, Mark and colleagues[6] observed labyrinthine signal changes in gadolinium chelate (GdC)-enhanced MRI only in patients with sudden deafness and vertigo, but not in normal inner ears. In another human study, no uptake of GdC was detected in the inner ear fluids, despite using triple-dose intravenous administration and a 1.5-T scanner.[7] In rodents, Counter and colleagues[1] studied guinea pigs and visualized abundant uptake of Gd in the perilymph of both cochlea and vestibule after intravenous administration of 5 times the human dose of GdC (by weight) imaged with a 4.7-T scanner. Zou and colleagues[2] performed mouse inner ear MRI studies (4.7 T) and observed efficient uptake of GdC with loading peak of 80 to 100 minutes after intravenous delivery. Direct visualization of EH in guinea pig was first reported by Zou and colleagues[8,9] in 2000 and followed by Niyazov and colleagues[10] in 2001. The controversial reports in the human studies compared with animal results raised 3 questions: Was the magnetic field too low in the human study? Was the concentration of GdC applied in humans too low? Was the observation time after intravenous administration of GdC in humans too short?

Alternatively, intratympanic administration of GdC provided efficient loading of the contrast agent in the inner ear perilymph and reduced the risk for systemic toxicity. MRI showed clear uptake of GdC in the perilymph of both rodents and humans after intratympanic delivery.[2,11–13] Naganawa and colleagues[13,14] improved the image quality and showed EH in humans using a three-dimensional (3D) fluid-attenuated inversion recovery (FLAIR) sequence in a 3-T machine.

This article describes the novel approaches that have been recently undertaken to visualize the inner ear. These approaches allow assessment of disease within the inner ear and also to follow dynamics regarding either recovery or deterioration of the diseases. Five major steps have been taken in the development of the ability to visualize enhancement within the human inner ear. These steps represent examples of translational research (ie, the development of a method in animal studies followed by application of the method to the benefit of human beings). The first step was to show that inner ear compartments could be distinguished using GdC-enhanced MRI. In normal inner ears of guinea pigs, it was observed that intravenously administered high doses (Omniscan 0.5 mmol/mL, 3 mL/kg intravenously) of GdC loaded the perilymph, but not the endolymph.[1] The second step was to show that visualization of EH was possible in animal models with intravenously administered GdC.[9] In animals with experimental EH, bulging of the Reissner's membrane could be visualized and quantified.[9] The third step was to show that when GdC was placed into the middle ear, the contrast agent passed through the middle-inner ear barriers (the round-window membrane) and the inner ear could be visualized.[9,15] For the fourth, the optimal imaging time for humans was determined and was shown to be about 22 hours after application of the contrast agent into the tympanic cavity.[5] However, more details were missing regarding the time points between 24 hours. For the fifth, modification of the sequences was necessary to increase the contrast between endolymph and perilymph with the lowest concentration of GdC in the perilymph. These sequences included 3D real inversion recovery (3D-real IR), rapid acquisition with relaxation enhancement (RARE), and FLAIR.[11,13,16–18]

To date, more than 100 patients have been evaluated and the identification of EH is broadening into other disease entities besides Meniere's syndrome, including recurrent vertigo, sudden deafness, and even superior canal dehiscence syndrome among others.[19] The current challenges in inner ear imaging are to improve the delivery of contrast agent so that the concentration of GdC in the inner ear exceeds the detecting limit and to develop more sensitive sequences. Combination of intravenous and local deliveries might produce maximum delivery of contrast agents into the inner ear by passing through both the blood-perilymph barrier and middle-inner ear barriers with minimum systemic toxicity. Another approach would be the development of additional contrast agents, such as the more recently available super paramagnetic iron nanoparticles (SPION).

CONTRAST AGENTS AND THEIR POSSIBLE TOXICITY TO THE INNER EAR

MRI contrast agents are a group of contrast media used to improve the visibility of internal body structures in MRI. Most MRI contrast agents work through shortening the T1 (eg, Gd) or T2 (eg, iron oxide) relaxation time of protons located nearby. Reduction of T1 relaxation time results in a hypersignal, whereas reduced T2 relaxation time reduces both T2 and T2* signals. Contrast agents interact with adjacent protons to influence their signal characteristics and the effects are recorded as the longitudinal relaxivity (r1) and transverse relaxivity (r2). Higher r1 values result in brightening or enhancement of tissue signal and higher r2 values result in darkening. In T1 (longitudinal relaxation time)-weighted sequences, the high r1 values of GdC produce desirable bright positive contrast effects, but the r1 decreases rapidly in higher field strengths.[14] Another disadvantage of GdC is that they require micromolar concentrations for visualization, whereas molecular imaging requires sensitivities in the nanomolar range. For these reasons, efforts are being made to synthesize nanoparticulate contrast agents with high relaxivities that when tagged with biologic markers allow for imaging of cellular process in high-strength magnetic fields.[20,21] Some examples of these novel nanoparticles are liposomes or micelles that contain paramagnetic GdC, nanoparticles created from GdC, and SPIONs.[22–28]

GdC Contrast Agents

The most commonly used clinical contrast agents are paramagnetic GdC that have longitudinal relaxivity (r1) values ranging from 10 to 20/s/mM.[29] However, the commonly encountered hexahydrate $GdCl_3$ $6H_2O$ cannot be used as an MRI contrast agent because of its low solubility in water at the near neutral pH of the body. Free Gd (Gd^{3+} ions), for example, $GdCl_2(H_2O)_6]^+$, is toxic. Chelating the Gd is essential for biomedical applications. One representative chelating agent is H_5DTPA (diethylenetriaminepentaacetic acid). Chelation to the conjugate base of this ligand increases the solubility of the Gd^{3+} at the neutral pH of the body and still allows for the paramagnetic effect required for an MRI contrast agent. The $DTPA^{5-}$ ligand binds to Gd through 5 oxygen atoms of the carboxylates and 3 nitrogen atoms of the amines. A ninth binding site remains, which is occupied by a water molecule. The rapid exchange of this water ligand with bulk water is a major reason for the signal-enhancing properties of the chelate. Two structurally distinct categories of GdC are currently marketed:

(1) macrocyclic chelates (gadoterate, gadoteridol, or gadobutrol), in which the Gd^{3+} ion is caged in the reorganized cavity of the ligand, and (2) linear chelates (gadopentetate, gadobenate, gadodiamide, gadoversetamide, gadofosveset/MS325, and gadoxetate). GdC can also be nonionic (or neutral), in which the number of carboxyl groups is reduced to 3, neutralizing the 3 positive charges of the Gd^{3+}, or ionic, in which the remaining carboxyl groups are salified with meglumine or sodium.[30]

Table 1 shows the GdC contrast agents in general use.

Gadopentetate dimeglumine (Magnevist) is a formation composed of Gd^{3+} complexed with DTPA (Gd-DTPA). DTPA is a chelator that surrounds Gd^{3+}. It is reported that Gd-DTPA exists as free Gd in concentration of 10^{-22} mol/L if the number of free Gd and the chelator (DTPA) are maintained at the same concentrations. Gadodiamide is a formulation composed of Gd^{3+} complexed with DTPA bis-methylamide (Gd-DTPA-BMA). The DTPA remains a chelator that surrounds Gd^{3+} and BMA maintains the contrast medium in a nonionized state. It is reported that of Gd-DTPA-BMA, 10^{-17} mol/L exists as free Gd ions if the number of free Gd and the chelator (DTPA-BMA) are maintained at the same concentrations.

SPION

Two commercially available classes of iron oxide particles are used in MRI for detection of malignant tumors and metastatic disease. SPIONs are used to visualize liver metastases. The particles are phagocytized by hepatic macrophages in healthy tissue, but not in metastases, which are shown as bright lesions against the darkened normal background liver. An increase in signal intensity indicates altered capillary permeability in tumor. These specific signal changes are valuable for differentiating benign from malignant enlarged lymph nodes.[31–33]

SPIONs currently in clinical use have r2 values ranging from 50 to more than 600/s/mM[25,34] and the values are stable with increasing magnetic field strengths. Similar to GdC, the r1 values decrease with increasing field strength.[35] Thus, in high magnetic fields of 3.0 T or more, SPIONs retain their strong darkening effect on T2 (transverse relaxation time)-weighted sequences, which would be seen in contrast to the bright signal ordinarily detected in fluid spaces. SPIONs targeted for specific cell types may be useful for differential imaging of the cochlea cell types.

Table 1
GdC contrast agents

General Name	Commercial Name	Structure
Ionic contrast agents		
Gadopentetate dimeglumine	Magnevist	Gd-DTPA
Gadobenate dimeglumine	Multihance	Gd-BOPTA
Gadfosveset trisodium	Vasovist	Gd-DTPA-DPCP
Gadoxetate disodium	Primovist	Gd-EOB-DTPA
Gadoterate meglumine	Dotarem/Magnescope	Gd-DOTA
Nonionic contrast agents		
Gadobtrol	Gadovist	Gd-BT-DO3A
Gadodiamide	Omniscan	Gd-DTPA-BMA
Gadoteridol	Prohance	Gd-HP-DO3A
Gadoversetamide	Optimark	Gd-DTPA-BMEA

SPIONs incorporated into cationic liposomes decorated with antitransferrin receptor single-chain antibody fragment for lung metastasis showed bright enhancement in lung nodules on T2 MR imaging. It seems that complexed nanoparticle contrast agents may have significant alterations in relaxivity that could offer promising new opportunities for cellular imaging.[36]

TOXICITY OF GDC CONTRAST AGENT

GdC administered intratympanically distributes in the whole perilymph in 12 hours but disappears within 1 week.[13] It is important to evaluate how much GdC enters the perilymphatic space after intratympanic Gd administration. It is estimated that the concentration of GdC within the perilymph after the intratympanic administration of gadodiamide (Omniscan) diluted 8 times is 10^{-4} mol/L, which is a 5000-times dilution of the original gadodiamide.

Intravenously applied GdC moves into cochlear fluid space, especially into the perilymph. Following intravenous GdC administration, at the peak GdC concentration, the cochlear fluid is enhanced to a level similar to that in the cerebellum, which is estimated to be an 8000- to 16,000-times dilution of the injected GdC solution. It is estimated that the maximum GdC concentration in the inner ear achieved with the intratympanic administration of the 8-times dilution is similar to that achieved by the threefold GdC intravenous injection. Even after 2-fold GdC intravenous injection, it was possible to show EH in patients with Meniere's disease, although the GdC concentration in the perilymph was lower compared with that obtained after intratympanic GdC administration.

In cell cultures free Gd was toxic to isolated hair cells at a concentration of 10^{-5} mol/L (Jing Zou and Colleagues, unpublished data). Kakigi and colleagues[37] reported that intratympanically administered Gd-DTPA-BMA had adverse effects on the stria vascularis in guinea pigs. When Gd-DTPA-BMA was diluted 8 times, no adverse effect on the stria vascularis was observed. Kakigi and colleagues[37] also recorded reduction of endolymph potential and enlarged intercellular gap of intermediate cells in the cochleae at 60 minutes after receiving intratympanic administration of nondiluted Gd-DTPA-BMA, but not in the cochleae subjected to 8-times dilution of the contrast agent. Kimitsuki and colleagues[38] observed that free Gd blocked mechanoelectric transducer current in chick cochlear hair cells by decreasing the inward going mechanoelectric transducer currents, specifically the Ca^{2+} component. There were reports of Ca^{2+} channel activities and transient receptor potential channel vanilloid subfamily 4 expression in the stria vascularis.[39,40] However, Gd in Gd-DTPA-BMA behaves differently from free Gd ion.

The amount of GdC administered by intratympanic injection is less than 0.1% of that given by ordinary intravenous injection. Accordingly systemic adverse effects of the intratympanically delivered agent may be negligible, but adverse effects on the inner ear must be evaluated carefully. The mechanism is unknown regarding the interference of Gd-DTPA-BMA with endocochlear potential. Our preliminary study with 9 healthy guinea pigs after intratympanic administration of nondiluted Gd-DTPA-BMA did not show threshold shift in tone auditory brainstem response (Ilmari Pyykkö, MD and Jing Zou, MD, unpublished data acquired in Stockholm). However, the middle ear mucosa showed inflammatory changes.[11] In humans, Fukuoka and colleagues[19] injected 8-fold dilutions of Gd-DTPA-BMA intratympanically into the ears of the diseased side and the contralateral healthy side, but no adverse effects were observed, even in the healthy ears.

To avoid any complications with free Gd it is recommended to use GdC immediately after the package is opened. Once the package is opened, the free Gd concentration may increase, even if the solution is kept in a refrigerator.

To our knowledge, there has been no report of any adverse effect on the inner ear in humans after any GdC administration, even in patients with nephrogenic systemic fibrosis. Nephrogenic systemic fibrosis is the most serious complication caused by intravenous GdC administration. When GdC remains in the body for a long time, the chelator surrounding the Gd gradually separates and the toxicity of free Gd becomes apparent. Nephrogenic systemic fibrosis occurs in relation to renal diseases that prevent free Gd excretion from the body, therefore its use is not recommended in patients with impaired kidney function. The incidence of nephrogenic systemic fibrosis seems to depend on the type of the GdC contrast agent. Altun and colleagues[41] reported that nephrogenic systemic fibrosis was not observed with the application of Gd-DTPA or Gd-DOTA rather than Gd-DTPA-BMA. Gd-based contrast media may be nephrotoxic even at approved doses. The toxicity of free Gd to the inner ear should be further investigated from various perspectives.

APPLICATION OF CONTRAST AGENTS
Intravenous Delivery of GdC

To deliver the contrast agent, the most extensively applied approach is intravenous injection. Because of its molecular size, GdC does not pass through the normal blood-brain barrier, thus making it valuable by visualizing the leakage of GdC through a damaged blood-brain barrier in diseases. The inner ear biologic barrier system is similar to the brain in that GdC does not pass through the normal blood-endolymph barrier and causes enhancement when lesions to the barrier occur as a result of mechanical force and inflammation.[8,9,11,35–37] Because the cochlear compartments are separated by the Reissner's membrane and the basilar membrane, which limit the passage of GdC, the efficient passage of GdC through the blood-perilymph barrier highlights the scala tympani and scala vestibuli, but not the scala media. A shift of the border between the dark scala media and bright scala vestibuli or scala tympani indicates a volume change in the endolymph. EH was first shown by such alterations in GdC enhancement within the scala vestibuli by MRI in both animal models and Meniere's disease.[9,13] The dosage applied in animals was 1.5 mmol/kg and 0.2 mmol/kg to 0.3 mmol/kg in humans.[1,18,20] At lower doses, the concentration of contrast was insufficient to clearly separate endolymph from perilymph, even using 3D FLAIR sequences with an 8-channel coil and a 3-T magnet.[14] Some patients have been studied using double-dose intravenous Gd contrast and imaging with a 32-channel head coil at 3 T. In those patients with Meniere's disease, EH was successfully visualized, despite the concentration of Gd-DTPA tending to be lower than with an intratympanic injection of 8-fold diluted Gd (**Fig. 1**).[18] In comparison, the routine dosage of GdC in the clinic is 0.1 mmol/kg and the maximum dose approved by the US Food and Drug Administration is 0.3 mmol/kg.

Intratympanic Administration of GdC

Intratympanic administration of GdC can potentially induce higher concentrations of contrast agent into the perilymph than by intravenous administration.[42] There are 2 potential pathways for the MRI contrast agents to enter the inner ear from the tympanic cavity. One is the round-window membrane and the other is the annular ligament of the stapediovestibular joint.[11] The transport efficacy of substances through

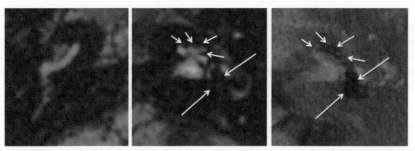

Fig. 1. A 36-year-old man with left Meniere's disease. 3D FLAIR (*left and middle image*) and 3D real IR image (*right image*) were obtained 4 hours after intravenous injection of double-dose Gd-DTPA. Dilated endolymphatic space was visualized in cochlea and vestibule of left labyrinth (*short and long arrows*). Vestibular endolymphatic space occupies almost all space, thus delineation of endolymphatic space of vestibule is clearer on 3D real IR than on 3D FLAIR (*long arrows*). EH was not seen in the right labyrinth (*left image*). The intravenous injection method enabled evaluation of both ears simultaneously.

these barriers may vary and depends on the size and surface characteristic of the particles and charge of the compounds.

Compounds may diffuse through the round-window membrane via paracellular pathways and extracellular matrix or by internalization via endocytosis (the process of uptake of macromolecules into cells by enclosing them in membrane vesicles). Three mechanisms are involved in pinocytosis: macropinocytosis, clathrin-mediated endocytosis, and caveolin-mediated endocytosis. In general, particles greater than 1 μm are internalized by macropinocytosis, particles with the size of around 120 nm are taken up by clathrin-mediated endocytosis, and 50- to 60-nm particles are internalized by caveolin-mediated endocytosis. Small and nonpolar molecules such as O_2 and CO_2 can readily diffuse across the lipid bilayer.[43] However, polar molecules such as Gd^{3+} ions are incapable of crossing the plasma membrane on their own. Gd^{3+} ions can be transported across the lipid bilayer through specialized membrane-transport Ca^{2+} channel by mimicking the properties of calcium.[44] Most other nanoscale molecular assemblies are internalized through endocytosis on contact with the cell membrane.[43] Ultrastructural studies of the round-window membrane of the cat showed that cationic ferritin, placed for 2 hours in the round-window niche of 4 normal cats, was observed to traverse the round-window membrane through pinocytotic vesicles into the connective tissue layer. Evidence of exocytosis of tracer by the inner epithelial layer into the scala tympani was presented. When placed in perilymph, this same tracer was incorporated by inner epithelial cells, suggesting transmembrane trafficking properties of the round-window membrane.[45]

Intratympanic delivery of GdC allows for efficient visualization of the cochlear compartments in both animals and humans.[2,11,13] GdC, diluted 5-fold, was optimal for imaging the animal cochlear compartments and diluted 8-fold was reasonable for imaging the cochlear scalae in humans.[2,13] GdC has been delivered to the round-window membrane by injection through the tympanic membrane, by topical application of gelatin sponge, or by installation of a cannula in the middle ear or bulla.[2,11–13] Transtympanic injection is the least traumatic and is as efficient as the gelatin sponge technique, making it more practical for clinical application.[46]

In humans GdC has been delivered into the middle ear by transtympanic injection. Two tiny spots (1 mm) on the tympanic membrane (one in the hypotympanic part, the other facing the Eustachian tube orifice) were topically anesthetized with 90% phenol solution (**Fig. 2**). A small hole in the tympanic membrane was made by the needle in the anesthetized anterior-superior spot to vent air during the injection. Through a 22-G needle, 0.5 mL of Gd contrast agent was injected through the hypotympanic spot into the middle ear cavity. The patient was kept recumbent with the treated diseased ear up for 15 to 30 minutes. Thereafter, the patient was allowed to move freely.

MRI TECHNIQUES OF INNER EAR
Animal Experiments

MRI parameters
In animal imaging a Bruker Biospec Avance 47/40 experimental MRI system with a magnetic field strength of 4.7 T and a 40-cm bore is commonly used (Bruker Medizintechnik, Karlsruhe-Ettlingen, Germany). Scanners are now available for animal use with even higher magnetic fields, such as 9.4 T. However, limited imaging depths and altered visualization of contrast agents with these stronger magnets make them less practical for rodents. The uptake of GdC in the guinea pig cochlear partitions was monitored in 10-min intervals for 40 to 90 minutes following administration. This strategy allowed for the generation of images with 100 averages for each evaluation point. The field of view was 3 cm, slice thickness 0.5 mm, center-center separation 0.65 mm, acquisition matrix 256 * 256 and reconstruction matrix 512 * 512, recovery time 500 ms, and repetition time 693.1 ms. RARE factor was 32, time between refocusing pulses 6.1 ms and phase encoding gradient increment, such as to yield an effective echo time of 31.5 ms. The parameters in depth are explained in detail elsewhere.[11]

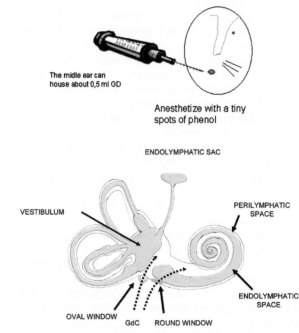

Fig. 2. Topical delivery of GdC with 2-hole technique (*top*). Pathways and barriers for GdC passage to the cochlea and vestibular system (*bottom*).

An advantage of two-dimensional MRI is that symmetric images can be made for comparison between left and right sides. However, some finer structures may not be delineated. Therefore 3D imaging with high-resolution T1-weighted RARE sequences (TR/TE$_{eff}$ 500/43 ms, RARE factor 16, matrix size 64 × 64 × 64, field of view 0.5 cm, resolution 0.078 × 0.078 × 0.078 mm^3, number of averages 2) are useful and showed delicate cochlear structures, even within the small inner ear of the mouse **(Fig. 3).**[2]

Visualizing an experimental animal inner ear

The modiolus, a potential communication site for perilymph, can be divided into a neural region and a vascular region. The vascular region communicates with the perilymph of both scala tympani and scala vestibuli.[47] This information is important for understanding the pathways of contrast agent in the cochlea.

After intravenous delivery, the GdC uptake in the guinea pig inner ear proceeded in the following order: first, GdC was detected in the modiolus and the area around the eighth nerve within 10 minutes; second, the scala tympani revealed substantial GdC uptake between 10 and 20 minutes; and third, GdC was measured in the scala vestibuli within 30 minutes and was nondetectable in the scala media by 90 minutes **(Fig. 4).**[15,47] The greatest and most rapid uptake was localized around the eighth nerve and modiolus. The modiolus within the basal turn and scala tympani in the second turn revealed significantly higher GdC uptake than in the other turns.[15] Intravenously applied GdC reached the scala tympani faster than the scala vestibuli. The modiolus within the third turn seemed brighter than in the other locations.[15,47]

After transtympanic delivery, GdC filled the basal turn within 40 minutes. Within 10 minutes after administration, GdC showed uptake in the outer point of the basal turn of

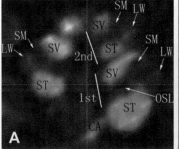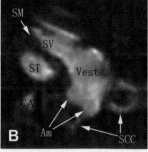

Fig. 3. Mouse inner ear structures in multiplanar reconstruction mono view of 3D T1-weighted images with IT administration of Gd-DOTA (23-mm coil) (3 hours). Gelfoam soaked with 5 μl, 500 mmol/L Gd-DOTA was placed into the left ear. (A) Cochlea. LW and Mod are slightly highlighted by Gd-DOTA uptake in addition to more pronounced enhancement in ST and SV. The structure adjacent to ST is suspected to be CA with signal intensity similar to ST. LW showed brighter signal than SM. A dark border appeared between ST and LW in the basal turn near the hook region. OSL is seen as a sharp dark line. (B) Vestibule. Gd-DOTA uptake was detected in the perilymph of Vest, Am, and SCC. The perilymph in the Vest merges with the perilymph in the basal turn of SV. CA is seen below the basal turn of the ST. Am, ampulla; CA, cochlear aqueduct; LW, lateral wall; OSL, osseous spiral lamina; SCC, semicircular canal; SM, the scala media; ST, the scala tympani; SV, the scala vestibuli; Vest, vestibulum; 1st, the basal turn; 2nd, the second turn. (*Adapted from* Zou J, Zhang W, Poe D, et al. Differential passage of gadolinium through the mouse inner ear barriers evaluated with 4.7T MRI. Hear Res 2010;259(1–2):37; with permission.)

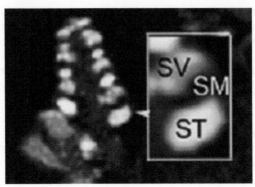

Fig. 4. Differential uptake of Gd in the guinea pig cochlear scalae at 90 minutes after intravenous injection. No entry of Gd into the scala media. SM, scala media; ST, scala tympani; SV, scala vestibuli.

the scala tympani and scala vestibuli (**Fig. 5**). Twenty minutes after administration, GdC appeared in the inner point of the scala vestibuli of the basal turn. Thirty minutes after administration, the intensity of GdC in the scala vestibuli of the basal turn was higher than that in the scala tympani. Within 60 minutes from administration the GdC reached the apex (helicotrema) of the cochlea. GdC appeared in the horizontal semicircular canal ampulla 10 minutes after transtympanic administration and showed uptake in the whole horizontal semicircular canal by 30 minutes.[11,47]

MRI of the mouse inner ear is desirable because the genome of the mouse is closer to humans' than is the guinea pig's and more biologic models and methodologies are available for the mouse. Consequently, we recently established GdC-enhanced MRI methods for the mouse inner ear.[2] We have successfully visualized GdC uptake into perilymph following intravenous and intratympanic administration.[2] As **Fig. 3** shows,

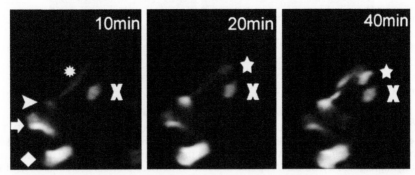

Fig. 5. Dynamic distribution of Gd-DTPA-BMA in the guinea pig cochlea after intratympanic administration showing the radial pathway through the modiolus and lateral wall. Ten minutes after administration, Gd appeared in the semicircular canal (*white arrow*), scala tympani (*white diamond*) of the basal turn, a minor amount in the scala vestibuli (*white asterisk*), the vascular region of modiolus (*white cross*), and the other end of the scala tympani (*white arrowhead*). Forty minutes later, a greater amount of contrast agent was visible in the vasculature region of the modiolus, the other end of the scala tympani, and scala vestibuli (*white star*). (*Adapted from* Zou J, Pyykko I, Bjelke B, et al. Communication between the perilymphatic scalae and spiral ligament visualized by in vivo MRI. Audiol Neurootol 2005;10(3):147.)

GdC uptake was visualized in the perilymph of both cochlear scalae and vestibule after intratympanic delivery.

Visualizing EH in animal experiments

To obtain precise information on the correlation of MRI and pathologic changes, animal models are relevant because the disease conditions can be well controlled. Several models have been developed to simulate human inner ear diseases, and their manifestations in MRI have been reported. These manifestations are shear stress (mechanical vibration), noise-induced hearing loss, immunoreaction-induced EH, and endolymphatic sac isolation-induced EH (Zou's model).[8,9,48–51]

Zou's model is less aggressive and simulates Meniere's disease better than Kimura's model by gently dissecting the endolymphatic sac from the sigmoid sinus and covering its outer surface with tissue sealant.[8,9,52,53] In Zou's model, the endolymphatic sac was kept intact but defunctionalized, and experimental EH could be visualized during the acute stage (6 days after operation) with 4.7-T MRI in vivo using intravenously delivered GdC.[8,9] The stria vascularis was impermeable to GdC during this stage and did not pass GdC to the endolymphatic compartment (scala media) from the GdC-contrasted perilymphatic compartments (scala vestibuli and scala tympani) in RARE images. The GdC-enhanced 4.7-T MRI showed enlarged endolymph space in the scala media, because endolymph partly displaced the perilymph in the scala vestibule. The respective findings were confirmed in histology, which showed typical EH.[8,9] Severe damage to the inner ear barrier with GdC leakage into the scala media was detected with MRI in an animal showing 60 dB hearing loss during chronic process of the pathologic change.[9]

Potentially, the immunoreaction-induced EH simulates Meniere's disease and other inner ear diseases better than the surgical models.[54] We have evaluated MRI in aseptic delayed EH by challenging the middle ear of guinea pig with keyhole limpet hemocyanin (KLH).[51] The MRI with intravenous delivery of GdC showed interesting changes: a disruption of the blood-endolymph barrier and development of EH (Fig. 6).[51] Increased uptake of GdC in the perilymph of both scala vestibuli and scala tympani occurred 30 minutes after contrast agent administration. The uptake in endolymph was obvious at 50 minutes after the GdC delivery. The change in the blood-perilymph barrier was greater than in the blood-endolymph barrier. This finding indicated that the mechanism of EH mediated by immunoreaction is different from that of endolymphatic sac dysfunction-induced EH, and blood-endolymph barrier disruption may be one of the mechanisms of EH in humans that can be assessed with MRI.[9,51]

MRI of Inner Ear in Humans

MRI sequences to visualize EH

For imaging the inner ear, high spatial resolution is mandatory. To visualize anatomy of the labyrinth heavily T2-weighted hydrography[55] or contrast-enhanced images[13,56] have been used. MR hydrography using heavily T2-weighted imaging showed high signal-to-noise ratio (SNR) even at lower static magnetic field such as 0.35 T[57]; however, a contrast-enhanced scan such as 3D FLAIR suffers from poor SNR at lower magnetic field than 3 T.[14] To increase SNR, there are 2 practical ways: one is to use the optimized receiver coil for signal reception; the other is to use a higher magnetic field.

Inner ear MRI using surface coil for signal reception has been reported from an early stage of clinical MRI. In adult humans, 8- to 12-cm-diameter circular coil was initially used to image the unilateral ear, because the depth sensitivity of the coil is typically the

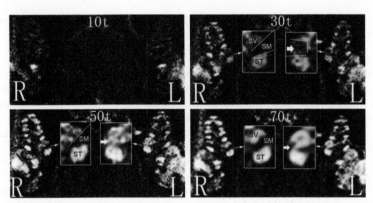

Fig. 6. MRI manifestation of KLH middle ear immunoreaction-induced EH. At the time window of 30 minutes, evident EH was shown in the cochlea from the basal to the apical turns. Significant uptake of Gd-DTPA-BMA in the scala media of the basal turn was shown at the 50-minute time window. The membranous lateral wall and spiral lamina, which is in continuous with the organ of Corti, are distinguished from the endolymph and perilymph by a dark image at the 70-minute time window. 10 t, 10 minutes after Gd-DTPA-BMA injection intravenously. (*Adapted from* Zou J, Pyykkö I, Börje B, et al. In vivo MRI visualization of endolymphatic hydrops induced by keyhole limpet hemocyanin round window immunization. Audiol Med 2007;5:185; with permission.)

same as half of its diameter. Later, phased-array technology enabled the simultaneous use of bilateral surface coils, and furthermore each side became quadrature in design to increase SNR.[3,58] High-resolution heavily T2-weighted MR cisternography using these phased-array quadrature coils made it possible to reliably screen an acoustic tumor in the internal auditory canal and cerebellopontine angle without GdC contrast.[3]

After the development of the parallel imaging technique using multiple-channel receiver coils,[59] which permit the acceleration of the speed of the MR scan, a multichannel phased-array head coil such as 8-channel or 12-channel became popular. To cover the whole brain and to permit parallel imaging in any desired plane, coil just covering the ears is insufficient for clinical neuroimaging. More recently a 32-channel phased-array head coil has become commercially available and permits high SNR covering the whole brain.[60]

The method for inner ear imaging was adapted from MR cisternography that sacrifices the soft-tissue contrast to achieve high spatial resolution of free water, which has a long T2 relaxation time. Endolymph and perilymph fluids in the labyrinth also showed bright signal as well as cerebrospinal fluid (CSF) in the cistern. Fine anatomy of the inner ear and disease was visualized as filling defects in water. There are 2 types of image acquisition methods for MR cisternography.[61] One is 3D fast spin-echo (3D FSE)-based techniques. In this group there are many varieties of techniques, such as fast recovery 3D FSE or turbospin echo (TSE),[62] sampling perfection with application optimized contrasts using different flip angle evolutions,[63,64] driven equilibrium radio frequency reset pulse,[65] volume isotropic T2-weighted acquisition, and extended echo-train acquisition.[66] Steady-state free precession-based techniques include CISS,[61] fast imaging employing steady state acquisition,[67] and balanced fast field echo.[68] Steady-state free precession-based techniques have a higher SNR than 3D FSE-based techniques; however, they have susceptibility artifacts.[61,68] The MR cisternography technique at 3 T visualizes the internal anatomy of the labyrinth such as the macula utriculi, macula sacculi, and crista ampullaris.[55] MR cisternography is also important for setting the anatomic reference for endo-/perilymphatic imaging,[69] because MR cisternography shows endo- and perilymphatic fluid spaces as high signal simultaneously.

Visualization of EH in humans has been tried previously by many researchers,[10,70,71] but it was not achieved in vivo until around 2005 to 2007.[11,13] There are several ways to separately visualize the endo-/perilymph fluid. The current method is based on the fact that the endolymphatic space is protected or isolated from perilymph, CSF, and blood. It uses the differences in the barriers for endo- and perilymph. In animals and humans, round-window application of GdC induced enhancement only of perilymph, not endolymph.[11] To minimize the adverse effect of GdC, contrast agent was diluted with saline. However, dilution of contrast media requires a highly sensitive imaging sequence. A FLAIR sequence is sensitive to various subtle T1 changes or subtle compositional alterations of fluid.[14,72] To achieve high SNR and thin slice, 3D FLAIR is used, and EH in patients with Meniere's disease can be visualized.[13] 3D FLAIR showed GdC containing perilymph as high signal and endolymph without GdC distribution and surrounding bone as zero signal (black). Therefore, sometimes it was difficult to delineate the endolymphatic space surrounded by bone. To separate endolymph, perilymph, and bone on a single image, 3D real IR was used.[16] 3D real IR allows separation of the positive and negative longitudinal magnetization. By shortening the inversion time from that of 3D FLAIR, GdC containing perilymph has positive magnetization, endolymph and CSF have negative magnetization, and bone with no proton has zero magnetization by 3D real IR (**Fig. 7**). The 3D real IR technique, however, is not so sensitive to low concentration of GdC as 3D FLAIR,[17,21] and so 3D FLAIR is still necessary.

For the extensive use of EH imaging, the MRI technique should be simpler. In a few cases, imaging at 1.5 T has been performed and succeeded in visualizing EH by intratympanic injection. Some MR scanners do not have the capability for a proper 3D FLAIR setting or 3D real IR setting. Those patients can be scanned by 2D FLAIR, with successful results.

Imaging of EH in humans

Classification of EH in MRI In the criteria of the 1995 AAO-HNS, certain, definite, probable, and possible Meniere's disease was defined. According to our experience of inner ear imaging in more than 100 ears, EH was shown in almost all patients with definite and probable Meniere's disease. In possible Meniere's disease with episodic

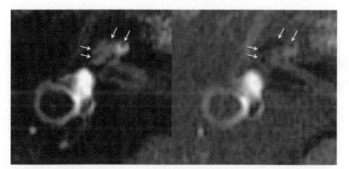

Fig. 7. A 33-year-old man with right-side Meniere's disease. 3D FLAIR (*left*) and 3D real IR (*right*) image obtained 24 hours after intratympanic injection of 8-fold diluted Gd-DTPA. Enlarged endolymphatic space (*arrows*) is prominent especially in cochlea. The border between the endolymphatic space (cochlear duct) and surrounding bone is not clear on 3D FLAIR.

vertigo of the Meniere's type without hearing loss, there were patients with and without EH in MRI.

Because endolymphatic space imaging has started to be used or is being planned in many hospitals, standardization of the evaluation of EH in MRI is necessary. A simple 3-stage grading of EH in the vestibule and the cochlea has been proposed (the 2008 Nagoya scale).[73] This scale is shown in **Table 1**. Further advancement in MRI is expected to allow more detailed imaging and classification. When the grade of EH differs between the basal and apical turns, we recommend reporting the highest grade of EH in the cochlea for this individual **Table 2**.

In MRI, the cochlear endolymphatic space is divided into cochlear turns, and each space is small. However, the section that includes the modiolus (midmodiolar section) is the most suitable region for evaluating the endolymphatic space. Not only the midmodiolar section but also other sections that include the cochlea are useful in the evaluation of the endolymphatic space in the cochlea. However, it is occasionally difficult to evaluate the endolymphatic space in all cochlear turns.

In the vestibule, when the area ratio of endolymphatic space to the vestibular fluid space exceeds one-third, it is judged as EH. When the endolymphatic space exceeds 50% of the fluid area in the vestibule, it is classified as significant hydrops. In temporal bone specimens from patients without inner ear diseases, the area ratio of endolymphatic space to the vestibular fluid ranged from 26.5% to 39.4% (mean 33.2%). **Fig. 8** shows a sac-operated patient with long duration of Meniere's disease and prominent EH in cochlea and vestibule.

When there is collapse of the endolymphatic space, it is not possible to distinguish the endolymphatic leakage of GdC from the rupture of Reissner's membrane in MRI scans. Moreover, if there is rupture of the Reissner's membrane, GdC may enter the endolymphatic space. Collapse of the endolymphatic space in the cochlea was suspected in one patient, and collapse of the endolymphatic space in the vestibule was suspected in another patient. In one patient with large vestibular aqueduct syndrome, rupture of the Reissner's membrane was suspected after deterioration in their hearing level. In this patient, GdC was seen in the endolymph of the endolymphatic sac and duct. Accordingly, classification as no hydrops does not always mean normal. In animal models ruptures could be visualized in histologic specimens, and in MRI rapid leakage of GdC into the scala media was seen, supporting the idea of intracochlear ruptures in Meniere's disease. Nevertheless, when the technique of visualizing the inner ear with intravenous contrast agent delivery is available these shortcomings

---

Table 2
Grading of EH using MRI

Grade of Hydrops	Vestibule (Area Ratio[a]) (%)	Cochlea
None	≤33.3	No displacement of Reissner's membrane
Mild	>33.3	Displacement of Reissner's membrane
	≤50	Area of cochlear duct ≤ area of the scala vestibuli
Significant	>50	Area of the cochlear duct exceeds the area of the scala vestibuli

[a] Ratio of the area of the endolymphatic space to that of the fluid space (sum of the endolymphatic and perilymphatic spaces) in the vestibule measured on tracings of images.

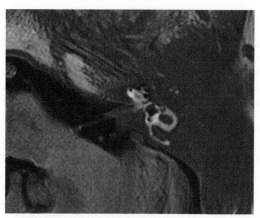

Fig. 8. Prominent EH in endolymphatic sac-operated patients. Note especially at the apex of cochlea the enlarged endolymphatic space and in the vestibulum and crista of the semicircular canals the hydropic displacement of GdC-filled perilymph.

with the intratympanic application technique can be solved. **Fig. 9** shows GdC movement into the endolymphatic sac from the perilymph in a patient with large vestibular aqueduct syndrome. The imaging was performed 4 days after acute deterioration of hearing level. MRI before and after intratympanic GdC administration revealed that the GdC entered the endolymphatic sac probably through the ruptured Reissner's membrane (see **Fig. 9**).

Time window for imaging In humans, GdC did not reach the apical turn of the cochlea when 7 hours passed after intratympanic injection.[13] It was reported that GdC was observed in all locations of the inner ear when 12 hours passed after intratympanic GdC injection.[11] However, this finding could not be confirmed in another study that showed that GdC filled the basal turn and the vestibule after 2 hours and disappeared in the cochlea after 12 hours.[11] One day after intratympanic injection, GdC appeared in

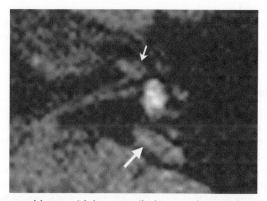

Fig. 9. MRI in a 27-year-old man with large vestibular aqueduct syndrome. The patient experienced acute hearing deterioration of left hearing level with vertigo. MRI was taken 1 day after intratympanic GdC injection. Compared with MRI taken before GdC injection, GdC enhancement was recognized in the enlarged endolymphatic duct and sac (*long arrow*). Short arrow indicates the cochlea.

CSF in the fundus area of the internal auditory canal.[74] Thus, GdC in the perilymph is absorbed not only through the modiolus and lateral wall of the cochlea but also through the CSF of the internal auditory canal. Six days after the intratympanic injection, GdC had almost disappeared from the inner ear.[13]

GdC administered intravenously also entered the perilymphatic space. Four hours after the intravenous GdC administration, the perilymphatic GdC concentration was at the highest level.[14,20] EH was observed in MRI taken 4 hours after double-dose GdC was injected intravenously.[18]

In 8 patients with fluctuating hearing loss without vertigo, EH was observed both in the cochlea and in the vestibule in all patients.[75] These cases were considered similar to Meniere's disease in MRI, although they were not defined as having probable or possible Meniere's disease according to the 1995 AAO-HNS criteria. Among patients with fluctuating hearing loss without vertigo, however, we recently experienced a patient in whom EH was observed in the cochlea but not in the vestibule in MRI.

In ears with profound hearing loss, it is occasionally difficult to diagnose EH using functional tests such as electrocochleography and the glycerol test. In patients with contralateral delayed EH, MRI after intratympanic GdC injection showed EH even in ears with profound hearing loss.[21]

Reduction of EH could be observed when the MRI was performed twice or more, with alleviation of the symptom in patients with Meniere's disease.[76,77] Thus, visualization of EH gives a new aspect for understanding Meniere's disease and related diseases.

Another purpose of MRI after intratympanic GdC administration is to investigate the permeability of the round-window membrane and to observe drug distribution inside the inner ear.[21] Intratympanic gentamicin administration is now used widely in the treatment of intractable Meniere's disease, and intratympanic steroid administration is used to treat sudden sensory hearing loss. Intratympanic drug administration therapy depends on the permeability of the round-window membrane. However, the permeability of the round-window membrane is diminished or poor in 13% of patients.[42] Confirming that an intratympanically applied drug reaches the inner ear and investigating its distribution inside the inner ear give useful information for intratympanic pharmaceutical therapy. In patients with large EH in the vestibule, the drug movement toward the semicircular canal is often disturbed because the route through the perilymphatic space is restricted in the vestibule because of the extended endolymphatic space.[21]

We believe that visualization of EH may be vital for making a new diagnosis of Meniere's disease. Investigation of the relationship between the endolymphatic image and development and severity of symptoms may deepen our understanding of inner ear diseases.

Future Expectations

Intratympanic administration of GdC is off-label and requires puncture of the tympanic membrane. To evaluate both ears simultaneously, it is necessary to inject GdC into both sides. These drawbacks hinder the development of this procedure. If intravenous injection of GdC could visualize EH, it would be convenient.

An uptake of the contrast agent in the scala media may indicate damage to the inner ear membranes, or possibly rupture of the Reissner's membrane, which was observed in one patient. It seems likely that local delivery can solve some of the imaging problems such as identification of EH or membrane rupture. Some disorders in animal models can be visualized only in intravenous delivery such as those linked to loading of GdC in the scala media. These disorders seem to indicate damage in the strial marginal and intermediate cells. Imaging of these changes is a challenge but the

Table 3
Inner ear disease with MRI with different application routes of contrast agent used for visualizing different nature of the disorder

Disease	Membranous Labyrinth Injury	Delivery Route of Gd
Meniere's disease	Reissner's membrane bulging or rupture	Transtympanic delivery/ intravenous delivery
Inner ear immune disorder	Stria vascularis disease/EH	Intravenous delivery or intratympanic delivery
Circulatory disturbances	Stria vascularis disease	Intravenous delivery
Spontaneous membrane rupture	Reissner's membrane	Intravenous delivery or intratympanic delivery
Perilymphatic fistula	Round-window membrane rupture or semicircular canal injury	Intravenous delivery or intratympanic delivery
Trauma	Stria vascularis disease	Intravenous delivery

development of novel contrast agents, coil technology and imaging sequences may solve this problem.

Direct visualization of the Reissner's membrane is straightforward. However, it has not been possible in living humans using a clinical MR unit because of limited resolution with the current magnetic field strength of maximum 3 T. Higher magnetic field strengths than 3 T might present some hazards to the human body. Another approach is to use the difference in sodium concentration in endo- and perilymph. Sodium MRI is possible at high field strength, such as 7 T; however, high-resolution sodium imaging for the inner ear is not practical even at 7 T because of its low SNR.

It is also possible to decrease the systemic loading of GdC by simultaneous intratympanic and intravenous injection to reach a higher inner ear/body ratio of the contrast agent. Both the blood-perilymph barrier and middle-inner ear barriers were used to transport the contrast agent. Potential disease of the blood-endolymph barrier can also be evaluated.

One of our nanoear partners has recently created a novel type of SPION in which the normally hydrophobic iron oxide nanoparticles are coated with a layer of oleic acid and covered with a surface layer of Pluronic F127 copolymer (PF127) to make the resultant 92-nm-diameter nanoparticles water soluble. This characteristic is desirable for medical applications to develop multifunctional contrast-agent nanoparticles for targeting the inflammatory molecules.[78,79] The targets include complement activation (C1q) and interleukin 1. Potentially, functionalized nanoparticles with binding peptides of these targets may also interfere with the process of Meniere's disease **Table 3**.

SUMMARY

In animal MRI experiments, both intravenous and intratympanic administration of Gd showed contrast agent uptake in the perilymph of the intact inner ear. The cochlear modiolus is the critical site for secreting perilymph and communicating perilymph between the scala tympani and scala vestibuli. Modiolar and spiral ligament pathways transport contrast agent to the vestibulum without passing the helicotrema. Intense noise exposure and immunoreaction-induced cochlear injury accelerated GdC passage though the blood-perilymph barrier. The blood-endolymph barrier was disrupted to leak GdC when the cochlea was exposed to intense noise and immune reaction. In humans, immediate GdC uptake in the inner ear perilymph was observed only in the impaired ear when administered intravenously. Intratympanic delivery of GdC showed higher signal-to-noise images of perilymphatic uptake in most patients with sensorineural hearing loss and Meniere's disease. MRI was also capable of showing EH in both animal models and patients with Meniere's disease. High-concentration GdC may affect the auditory physiology and should be further evaluated.

REFERENCES

1. Counter SA, Bjelke B, Klason T, et al. Magnetic resonance imaging of the cochlea, spiral ganglia and eighth nerve of the guinea pig. Neuroreport 1999; 10(3):473–9.
2. Zou J, Zhang W, Poe D, et al. Differential passage of gadolinium through the mouse inner ear barriers evaluated with 4.7T MRI. Hear Res 2010;259(1–2): 36–43.
3. Naganawa S, Ito T, Fukatsu H, et al. MR imaging of the inner ear: comparison of a three-dimensional fast spin-echo sequence with use of a dedicated quadrature-surface coil with a gadolinium-enhanced spoiled gradient-recalled sequence. Radiology 1998;208(3):679–85.
4. Teranishi M, Yoshida T, Katayama N, et al. 3D computerized model of endolymphatic hydrops from specimens of temporal bone. Acta Otolaryngol Suppl 2009;560:43–7.
5. Committee on Hearing and Equilibrium guidelines for the diagnosis and evaluation of therapy in Meniere's disease. American Academy of Otolaryngology-Head and Neck Foundation, Inc. Otolaryngol Head Neck Surg 1995;113(3):181–5.
6. Mark AS, Seltzer S, Nelson-Drake J, et al. Labyrinthine enhancement on gadolinium-enhanced magnetic resonance imaging in sudden deafness and vertigo: correlation with audiologic and electronystagmographic studies. Ann Otol Rhinol Laryngol 1992;101(6):459–64.
7. Naganawa S, Koshikawa T, Nakamura T, et al. High-resolution T1-weighted 3D real IR imaging of the temporal bone using triple-dose contrast material. Eur Radiol 2003;13(12):2650–8.
8. Zou J PI, Börje B, Bretlau P, et al. Endolymphatic hydrops is caused by increased porosity of stria vascularis [abstract]? Paper presented at Barany Society Meeting. Uppsala, Sweden, June 4–7, 2000.
9. Zou J, Pyykko I, Bretlau P, et al. In vivo visualization of endolymphatic hydrops in guinea pigs: magnetic resonance imaging evaluation at 4.7 tesla. Ann Otol Rhinol Laryngol 2003;112(12):1059–65.
10. Niyazov DM, Andrews JC, Strelioff D, et al. Diagnosis of endolymphatic hydrops in vivo with magnetic resonance imaging. Otol Neurotol 2001;22(6):813–7.
11. Zou J, Pyykko I, Bjelke B, et al. Communication between the perilymphatic scalae and spiral ligament visualized by in vivo MRI. Audiol Neurootol 2005;10(3): 145–52.
12. Duan M, Bjelke B, Fridberger A, et al. Imaging of the guinea pig cochlea following round window gadolinium application. Neuroreport 2004;15(12):1927–30.
13. Nakashima T, Naganawa S, Sugiura M, et al. Visualization of endolymphatic hydrops in patients with Meniere's disease. Laryngoscope 2007;117(3):415–20.
14. Naganawa S, Komada T, Fukatsu H, et al. Observation of contrast enhancement in the cochlear fluid space of healthy subjects using a 3D-FLAIR sequence at 3 Tesla. Eur Radiol 2006;16(3):733–7.

15. Zou J, Pyykko I, Counter SA, et al. In vivo observation of dynamic perilymph formation using 4.7 T MRI with gadolinium as a tracer. Acta Otolaryngol 2003; 123(8):910–5.
16. Naganawa S, Satake H, Kawamura M, et al. Separate visualization of endolymphatic space, perilymphatic space and bone by a single pulse sequence; 3D-inversion recovery imaging utilizing real reconstruction after intratympanic Gd-DTPA administration at 3 Tesla. Eur Radiol 2008;18(5):920–4.
17. Naganawa S, Nakashima T. Cutting edge of inner ear MRI. Acta Otolaryngol Suppl 2009;560:15–21.
18. Nakashima T, Naganawa S, Teranishi M, et al. Endolymphatic hydrops revealed by intravenous gadolinium injection in patients with Meniere's disease. Acta Otolaryngol 2010;130:338–43.
19. Fukuoka H, Tsukada K, Miyagawa M, et al. Semi-quantitative evaluation of endolymphatic hydrops by bilateral intratympanic gadolinium-based contrast agent (GBCA) administration with MRI for Meniere's disease. Acta Otolaryngol 2010; 130:10–6.
20. Carfrae MJ, Holtzman A, Eames F, et al. 3 Tesla delayed contrast magnetic resonance imaging evaluation of Meniere's disease. Laryngoscope 2008;118(3): 501–5.
21. Nakashima T, Naganawa S, Katayama N, et al. Clinical significance of endolymphatic imaging after intratympanic gadolinium injection. Acta Otolaryngol Suppl 2009;560:9–14.
22. Frias JC, Williams KJ, Fisher EA, et al. Recombinant HDL-like nanoparticles: a specific contrast agent for MRI of atherosclerotic plaques. J Am Chem Soc 2004;126(50):16316–7.
23. Lipinski MJ, Amirbekian V, Frias JC, et al. MRI to detect atherosclerosis with gadolinium-containing immunomicelles targeting the macrophage scavenger receptor. Magn Reson Med 2006;56(3):601–10.
24. Glogard C, Stensrud G, Hovland R, et al. Liposomes as carriers of amphiphilic gadolinium chelates: the effect of membrane composition on incorporation efficacy and in vitro relaxivity. Int J Pharm 2002;233(1–2):131–40.
25. Wunderbaldinger P, Josephson L, Weissleder R. Crosslinked iron oxides (CLIO): a new platform for the development of targeted MR contrast agents. Acad Radiol 2002;9(Suppl 2):S304–6.
26. Lanza GM, Abendschein DR, Yu X, et al. Molecular imaging and targeted drug delivery with a novel, ligand-directed paramagnetic nanoparticle technology. Acad Radiol 2002;9(Suppl 2):S330–1.
27. Winter PM, Caruthers SD, Yu X, et al. Improved molecular imaging contrast agent for detection of human thrombus. Magn Reson Med 2003;50(2):411–6.
28. Shen T, Weissleder R, Papisov M, et al. Monocrystalline iron oxide nanocompounds (MION): physicochemical properties. Magn Reson Med 1993;29(5): 599–604.
29. Mathews VP, Caldemeyer KS, Ulmer JL, et al. Effects of contrast dose, delayed imaging, and magnetization transfer saturation on gadolinium-enhanced MR imaging of brain lesions. J Magn Reson Imaging 1997;7(1):14–22.
30. Idee JM, Port M, Dencausse A, et al. Involvement of gadolinium chelates in the mechanism of nephrogenic systemic fibrosis: an update. Radiol Clin North Am 2009;47(5):855–69, vii.
31. Pouliquen D, Le Jeune JJ, Perdrisot R, et al. Iron oxide nanoparticles for use as an MRI contrast agent: pharmacokinetics and metabolism. Magn Reson Imaging 1991;9(3):275–83.

32. Guimaraes R, Clement O, Bittoun J, et al. MR lymphography with superparamagnetic iron nanoparticles in rats: pathologic basis for contrast enhancement. AJR Am J Roentgenol 1994;162(1):201–7.

33. Bordat C, Sich M, Rety F, et al. Distribution of iron oxide nanoparticles in rat lymph nodes studied using electron energy loss spectroscopy (EELS) and electron spectroscopic imaging (ESI). J Magn Reson Imaging 2000;12(3):505–9.

34. Moffat BA, Reddy GR, McConville P, et al. A novel polyacrylamide magnetic nanoparticle contrast agent for molecular imaging using MRI. Mol Imaging 2003;2(4):324–32.

35. Sosnovik DE, Weissleder R. Emerging concepts in molecular MRI. Curr Opin Biotechnol 2007;18(1):4–10.

36. Freedman M, Chang EH, Zhou Q, et al. Nanodelivery of MRI contrast agent enhances sensitivity of detection of lung cancer metastases. Acad Radiol 2009;16(5):627–37.

37. Kakigi A, Nishimura M, Takeda T, et al. Effects of gadolinium injected into the middle ear on the stria vascularis. Acta Otolaryngol 2008;128(8):841–5.

38. Kimitsuki T, Nakagawa T, Hisashi K, et al. Gadolinium blocks mechano-electric transducer current in chick cochlear hair cells. Hear Res 1996;101(1–2):75–80.

39. Inui T, Mori Y, Watanabe M, et al. Physiological role of L-type Ca2+ channels in marginal cells in the stria vascularis of guinea pigs. J Physiol Sci 2007;57(5):287–98.

40. Zou J, Minasyan A, Keisala T, et al. Progressive hearing loss in mice with a mutated vitamin D receptor gene. Audiol Neurootol 2008;13(4):219–30.

41. Thomsen HS. Gadolinium-based contrast media may be nephrotoxic even at approved doses. Eur Radiol 2004;14(9):1654–6.

42. Yoshioka M, Naganawa S, Sone M, et al. Individual differences in the permeability of the round window: evaluating the movement of intratympanic gadolinium into the inner ear. Otol Neurotol 2009;30(5):645–8.

43. Verma A, Stellacci F. Effect of surface properties on nanoparticle–cell interactions. Small 2010;6(1):12–21.

44. Pillai S, Bikle DD. Lanthanum influx into cultured human keratinocytes: effect on calcium flux and terminal differentiation. J Cell Physiol 1992;151(3):623–9.

45. Goycoolea MV, Carpenter AM, Muchow D. Ultrastructural studies of the round-window membrane of the cat. Arch Otolaryngol Head Neck Surg 1987;113(6):617–24.

46. Zou J, Ramadan UA, Pyykkö I. Gadolinium uptake in the rat inner ear perilymph evaluated with 4.7 T MRI: a comparison between transtympanic injection and gelatin sponge-based diffusion through the round window membrane. Otol Neurotol 2010;31:637–41.

47. Zou J, Poe D, Bjelke B, et al. Visualization of inner ear disorders with MRI in vivo: from animal models to human application. Acta Otolaryngol 2009;560:22–31.

48. Zou J, Pyykkö I, Sutinen P, et al. MRI presentation of the blood-labyrinth barrier change after cochlea vibration trauma. Chinese Journal of Otology (Beijing) 2006;4(1):61–4.

49. Counter SA, Bjelke B, Borg E, et al. Magnetic resonance imaging of the membranous labyrinth during in vivo gadolinium (Gd-DTPA-BMA) uptake in the normal and lesioned cochlea. Neuroreport 2000;11(18):3979–83.

50. Zou J, Pyykkö I, Börje B. Preliminary study on in vivo visualization of keyhole limpet hemocyanin middle ear immunization induced endolymphatic hydrops by MRI. Chinese Journal of Otology (Beijing) 2005;3(3):200–2003.

51. Zou J, Pyykkö I, Börje B, et al. In vivo MRI visualization of endolymphatic hydrops induced by keyhole limpet hemocyanin round window immunization. Audiol Med 2007;5:182–7.
52. Kimura RS. Experimental blockage of the endolymphatic duct and sac and its effect on the inner ear of the guinea pig. A study on endolymphatic hydrops. Ann Otol Rhinol Laryngol 1967;76(3):664–87.
53. Kimura RS. Experimental pathogenesis of hydrops. Arch Otorhinolaryngol 1976; 212(4):263–75.
54. Tomiyama S. Development of endolymphatic hydrops following immune response in the endolymphatic sac of the guinea pig. Acta Otolaryngol 1992; 112(3):470–8.
55. Lane JI, Witte RJ, Bolster B, et al. State of the art: 3T imaging of the membranous labyrinth. AJNR Am J Neuroradiol 2008;29(8):1436–40.
56. Nakashima T, Naganawa S, Pyykko I, et al. Grading of endolymphatic hydrops using magnetic resonance imaging. Acta Otolaryngol 2009;129:5–8.
57. Naganawa S, Ito T, Iwayama E, et al. High-resolution MR cisternography of the cerebellopontine angle, obtained with a three-dimensional fast asymmetric spin-echo sequence in a 0.35-T open MR imaging unit. AJNR Am J Neuroradiol 1999;20(6):1143–7.
58. Naganawa S, Ito T, Iwayama E, et al. MR imaging of the cochlear modiolus: area measurement in healthy subjects and in patients with a large endolymphatic duct and sac. Radiology 1999;213(3):819–23.
59. Griswold MA, Jakob PM, Heidemann RM, et al. Generalized autocalibrating partially parallel acquisitions (GRAPPA). Magn Reson Med 2002;47(6):1202–10.
60. Wiggins GC, Triantafyllou C, Potthast A, et al. 32-channel 3 Tesla receive-only phased-array head coil with soccer-ball element geometry. Magn Reson Med 2006;56(1):216–23.
61. Naganawa S, Koshikawa T, Fukatsu H, et al. MR cisternography of the cerebello-pontine angle: comparison of three-dimensional fast asymmetrical spin-echo and three-dimensional constructive interference in the steady-state sequences. AJNR Am J Neuroradiol 2001;22(6):1179–85.
62. Naganawa S, Koshikawa T, Fukatsu H, et al. Fast recovery 3D fast spin-echo MR imaging of the inner ear at 3 T. AJNR Am J Neuroradiol 2002;23(2): 299–302.
63. Mugler JP 3rd, Bao S, Mulkern RV, et al. Optimized single-slab three-dimensional spin-echo MR imaging of the brain. Radiology 2000;216(3):891–9.
64. Naganawa S, Kawai H, Fukatsu H, et al. High-speed imaging at 3 Tesla: a technical and clinical review with an emphasis on whole-brain 3D imaging. Magn Reson Med Sci 2004;3(4):177–87.
65. Jung NY, Moon WJ, Lee MH, et al. Magnetic resonance cisternography: comparison between 3-dimensional driven equilibrium with sensitivity encoding and 3-dimensional balanced fast-field echo sequences with sensitivity encoding. J Comput Assist Tomogr 2007;31(4):588–91.
66. Gold GE, Busse RF, Beehler C, et al. Isotropic MRI of the knee with 3D fast spin-echo extended echo-train acquisition (XETA): initial experience. AJR Am J Roentgenol 2007;188(5):1287–93.
67. Sheth S, Branstetter BF, Escott EJ. Appearance of normal cranial nerves on steady-state free precession MR images. Radiographics 2009;29(4):1045–55.
68. Byun JS, Kim HJ, Yim YJ, et al. MR imaging of the internal auditory canal and inner ear at 3T: comparison between 3D driven equilibrium and 3D balanced fast field echo sequences. Korean J Radiol 2008;9(3):212–8.

69. Naganawa S, Sugiura M, Kawamura M, et al. Imaging of endolymphatic and perilymphatic fluid at 3T after intratympanic administration of gadolinium-diethylenetriamine pentaacetic acid. AJNR 2008;29(4):724–6.

70. Koizuka I, Seo R, Sano M, et al. High-resolution magnetic resonance imaging of the human temporal bone. ORL J Otorhinolaryngol Relat Spec 1991;53(6):357–61.

71. Koizuka I, Seo Y, Murakami M, et al. Micro-magnetic resonance imaging of the inner ear in the guinea pig. NMR Biomed 1997;10(1):31–4.

72. Naganawa S, Koshikawa T, Nakamura T, et al. Comparison of flow artifacts between 2D-FLAIR and 3D-FLAIR sequences at 3 T. Eur Radiol 2004;14(10):1901–8.

73. Nakashima T, Naganawa S, Pyykko I, et al. Grading of endolymphatic hydrops using magnetic resonance imaging. Acta Otolaryngol Suppl 2009;560:5–8.

74. Naganawa S, Satake H, Iwano S, et al. Communication between cochlear perilymph and cerebrospinal fluid through the cochlear modiolus visualized after intratympanic administration of Gd-DTPA. Radiat Med 2008;26(10):597–602.

75. Teranishi M, Naganawa S, Katayama N, et al. Image evaluation of endolymphatic space in fluctuating hearing loss without vertigo. Eur Arch Otorhinolaryngol 2009; 266(12):1871–7.

76. Miyagawa M, Fukuoka H, Tsukada K, et al. Endolymphatic hydrops and therapeutic effects are visualized in 'atypical' Meniere's disease. Acta Otolaryngol 2009;129(11):1326–9.

77. Sone M, Naganawa S, Teranishi M, et al. Changes in endolymphatic hydrops in a patient with Meniere's disease observed using magnetic resonance imaging. Auris Nasus Larynx 2010;37(2):220–2.

78. Qin J, Asempah I, Laurent S, et al. Injectable superparamagnetic ferrogels for controlled release of hydrophobic drugs. Adv Mater 2009;21(13):1354–7.

79. Qin J, Laurent S, Jo YS, et al. A high-performance magnetic resonance imaging T-2 contrast agent. Adv Mater 2007;19:1874–8.

Medical and Noninvasive Therapy for Meniere's Disease

Simon L. Greenberg, MB BS (Hons), FRACS,
Julian M. Nedzelski, MD, FRCSC*

KEYWORDS

- Meniere's • Medical Management • Gentamicin
- Steroid • Streptomycin

The exact pathogenesis of Meniere's disease (MD) remains unclear. As a result, modern therapy for MD aims to control the symptoms of the condition adequately to allow a good quality of life. In practice, the aim of treatment is to reduce the severity and frequency of the vertiginous attacks, to prevent the long-term gradual deterioration of hearing, and to lessen the tinnitus over time. Despite more than 150 years passing since Prosper Ménière initially described the syndrome that now bears his name,[1] little evidence exists to support many of the treatments commonly used today. Torok[2] published an exhaustive review of this subject based on 834 papers[2] published between 1951 and 1975. His review questions the validity of many of the suggested treatments for MD, highlighting that the clinical outcomes in these studies were essentially the same, whatever the modality of treatment used. A recent review of the literature by Coelho and Lalwani[3] in 2008 highlights that despite a further 24 years of medical research, many of Torak's criticisms remain relevant.

TREATMENT OF ACUTE EXACERBATIONS

Acute attacks of MD are characterized by acute rotational vertigo, transient fluctuations in hearing, tinnitus, and, in many, aural fullness. Typically patients feel unwell and in some instances experience dramatic diaphoresis. Initial management focuses on excluding other conditions that can present with some of the same symptoms, including vestibular neuronitis, migraine, cerebral vascular events, and rarely other central conditions, including multiple sclerosis and tumors. The diagnosis of MD may become more apparent with time as the fluctuating and episodic nature of the

Funding support: No specific funding has been provided to either author and no conflict of interest exists.

Department of Otolaryngology-Head and Neck Surgery, Sunnybrook Health Sciences Centre, University of Toronto, 2075 Bayview Avenue, Room M1 102, Toronto, Ontario M4N3M5, Canada

* Corresponding author.

E-mail address: julian.nedzelski@sunnybrook.ca

symptoms becomes more obvious. The acute management of a patient with known MD is mainly symptomatic. Although hospitalization is rarely required, intravenous fluids may be required in the emergency department. Vestibular suppressants can be used for symptomatic control, although they can delay patients' recovery by suppressing the adaptive response if used over a longer interval. More recently, corticosteroids have been advocated in this setting to help with the vertigo and hearing loss. However, the use of steroids in this context is unproved.

LOW-SALT DIET AND LIFESTYLE MODIFICATION

Classic treatment paradigms of MD often begin with salt restriction and lifestyle modification. Endolymphatic hydrops has long been proposed as being related to the pathogenesis of MD. Classically, it has been believed that a high-salt diet can influence the osmotic gradients in the inner ear, resulting in endolymphatic hydrops. Some patients (although not all) report that a salt binge seems to precipitate an acute episode of MD. On the other hand, the exact relationship between endolymphatic hydrops and MD remains controversial. Furthermore, some investigators have challenged the simple notion that salt restriction affects the fluid dynamics of the ear in ways that would significantly influence the degree of hydrops present.[4] Levels of recommended salt restriction vary but figures often quoted range from 2 g per 24 hours down to 1 g per 24 hours. This level of salt restriction can be limiting on patients' lifestyles and quality of life. Patients are instructed to avoid adding salt to food, pay close attention to food labeling, and avoid processed foods. The input of a dietician is often helpful. Effective compliance is difficult to maintain in the long-term for most patients. Given these side effects, no strong evidence exists to support the role of salt restriction alone in reducing the frequency or severity of symptoms from MD.

DIURETICS

Diuresis has been proposed as a treatment of MD since at least the 1930s.[5] Theoretically, diuresis reduces the amount of endolymphatic hydrops by reducing the extracellular fluids in the body. There are many different diuretics and almost all of them have been proposed as a potential treatment of MD. Hydrochlorothiazide is perhaps the most widely advocated, although furosemide and spirinolactone have their supporters. Despite their widespread use, no clear scientific evidence exists to support their efficacy. A recent Cochrane review[6] found "there is no good evidence for or against the use of diuretics in MD."

BETAHISTINE

Cochlear vascular insufficiency as a result of autonomic dysfunction has been proposed as a cause of MD. As a result, betahistine has been proposed as a treatment because of its theoretic vasodilatory effects on the blood supply to the inner ear.[7] The exact mechanism of action of betahistine in this setting is not known. Pharmacologic testing in animals has shown that the blood circulation in the striae vascularis of the inner ear improves, probably by means of a relaxation of the precapillary sphincters of the microcirculation of the inner ear.[8,9] In further animal pharmacologic studies, betahistine was found to have weak H_1-receptor agonistic and considerable H_3-antagonistic properties in the central nervous system and autonomic nervous system.[10] The clinical efficacy of betahistine has been the subject of several trials.[11–14] Individually, many of these trials found betahistine to be effective in reducing the frequency or severity of vertiginous episodes and to some extent helping with tinnitus.

No evidence exists to show betahistine helps with symptoms of hearing loss. A recent Cochrane review[15] examining the role of betahistine reported that although individual trials provided positive results, a large randomized controlled trial is required to clarify its clinical efficacy.

CORTICOSTEROIDS

The potential autoimmune cause of MD, and the recent use of transtympanic steroids to treat sudden sensorineural hearing loss, have stimulated interest in the use of steroids for the treatment of MD. In addition to a possible immune-modulating effect, recent studies have suggested that steroid perfusion can influence sodium and fluid dynamics in the inner ear because of their mineralocorticoid properties.[16,17] Potential advantages of steroid use include the low risk of complications and the potential beneficial effect on hearing (when compared with the risk of hearing loss with gentamicin therapy). This effect may be particularly advantageous for those patients with bilateral MD. Early studies investigating the role of steroids in MD showed promising results, although these studies lacked adequate control groups.[18,19] Silverstein and colleagues[20] were the first to perform a randomized double-blind trial in which injection of transtympanic steroid was compared with placebo injection of saline. Although the trial was limited by small numbers, no difference was found between the 2 groups with regards to vertigo control, hearing loss, or tinnitus levels. However, more recently, Garduno-Anaya and colleagues[21] performed a similar study and found a beneficial effect in the group treated with steroids. Boleas-Aguirre and colleagues[22] have reported the results of a large retrospective series (129 patients) treated with transtympanic steroids for MD. Results were not reported according to the 1995 American Academy of Otolaryngology-Head and Neck Surgery (AAO-HNS) guidelines but rather by using the Kaplan-Meier method. Using these reporting criteria, 91% of patients were classified as achieving acceptable vertigo control. The use of steroids in MD remains an area in which more research is required.

MISCELLANEOUS MEDICAL TREATMENTS

Various other medications have been proposed as being useful for the management of MD. Isosorbide, adenosine triphosphate, γ-globulin, urea, glycerol, lithium, and anticholinergics have all been proposed as beneficial therapies. Clear evidence is lacking for the efficacy of these treatments.

Hormonal manipulation has been reported as a potential treatment of MD. Andrews and colleagues[23] reported a series of 6 female patients who suffered exacerbations of their MD in relation to their menstrual cycle. These investigators proposed that fluctuations in fluid retention in association with hormonal changes in the body may be an underlying cause. Subsequently Price and colleagues[24] reported on a patient with MD related to the menstrual cycle whose symptoms were alleviated when she was started on leuprolide acetate, a drug that blocks normal sex-hormone production.

Innovar is an anesthetic agent comprised of droperidol and fentanyl. Although not widely used for this purpose, Innovar has a strong suppressive effect on the vestibular system. Gates[25] reported his experience using Innovar to treat 12 patients with intractable vertigo despite maximal medical therapy as an alternative to second-line surgical interventions. Innovar resulted in long-term control of vertigo in 58% of patients in this study, and the author outlined his practice of offering treatment with Innovar to all patients in his practice as an alternative to traditional surgical intervention. Gates reported several potential advantages compared with endolymphatic sac surgery, including lower cost, reduced risk to hearing, and faster patient recovery following treatment.

Hyperbaric oxygen therapy has also been proposed as a treatment of patients with MD.[26] The efficacy of this therapy is unproved.

EDUCATION, STRESS REDUCTION, HEARING AIDS, AND TINNITUS TRAINING

In addition to the pharmacologic treatments mentioned earlier, other measures can have a significant clinical benefit for the patient with MD. Education is an important part of the treatment of MD. MD is a chronic condition and can be debilitating for patients. In an effort to reduce the effect of this disease on their quality of life, it is important that patients understand the likely clinical course of their condition and required treatment paradigms. Appropriate information can help alleviate the frustration and depression many patients experience because of feelings of helplessness or the misunderstanding of treatment options. Yardley and Kirby[27] examined the role of vestibular rehabilitation and psychological therapies such as relaxation techniques and cognitive behavioral therapy in 360 patients with MD. These investigators found a significant improvement in patients' outcomes following this therapy. Hearing aids can be used to treat the hearing loss associated with MD. Potential problems related to fluctuating hearing can be overcome if patients are capable of self-programming their own aids.[28] Tinnitus therapy can help patients to cope better with this often-distressing symptom.

MENIETT DEVICE

The Meniett device (Medtronic, Jacksonville, FL, USA) is a minimally invasive, nondestructive therapy that is a new addition to the treatment paradigm for MD. The rationale for its use is based on the observation that pressure changes applied to the inner ear result in beneficial changes in the symptoms of patients with MD. Patients require a standard ventilation tube to be placed before use. The Meniett device applies pulses of pressure to the inner ear via the ventilation tube. A treatment cycle takes 5 minutes and is repeated 3 times a day. Several studies investigating the efficacy of this treatment have reported promising results.[29-33] No significant complications have been reported with its use. Gates and colleagues[29] reported that 67% of patients using the device in their trial reported either a complete or significant long-term improvement in their vertigo. Similarly, Mattox and Reichert[30] used the Meniett device as an alternative to second-line therapy when first-line medical therapy had failed. A total of 63% of patients required no further intervention (ie, second-line treatments) despite being followed for 3 years. In addition, those patients who failed to gain a benefit from the device did so early in therapy, thereby avoiding the potential frustration of a prolonged trial, only to find limited success. Dornhoffer and King followed 12 patients using the Meniett device for an average duration of 4 years.[31] Of these patients, 25% showed no benefit from the device, whereas 75% reported a reduction in the frequency and severity of their vertigo. Rajan and colleagues[32] analyzed 18 patients using the device and reported that 12 patients achieved a significant improvement in their vertigo and 5 patients showed improved hearing results. All 6 patients who did not respond to the Meniett device had been previously treated with gentamicin or surgery. These investigators propose that the efficacy of the Meniett device may be impaired by these previous treatments. Thomsen and colleagues[33] performed a randomized double-blind placebo-controlled study of the effect of the Meniett device. Patients were randomized into 2 groups. The first group used the Meniett device for 2 months. The placebo group was given a fake device that was indistinguishable from the true Meniett device. Forty patients entered the study. The study showed a reduction of the frequency of vertiginous attacks in those with the real device versus those with the placebo. However, this result was not statistically significant. Patient perception of the severity of the vertigo and the functionality level of the active group improved when compared with the placebo group, with results that were statistically significant. With respect to patient perception of hearing, tinnitus, and aural pressure, there was no significant difference between the groups. Although many of these studies reported positive findings, the numbers of patients in these studies is small and the efficacy of the Meniett device remains unclear.

TREATMENT WITH AMINOGLYCOSIDES

Despite various combinations and permutations of these treatment options, some patients persistently experience debilitating vertigo from their MD. For such patients, vestibulotoxic medication can be used to abolish or greatly reduce vestibular activity in the affected ear, hence alleviating symptoms of vertigo and potentially preserving hearing. Aminoglycosides are a family of antibiotics that are toxic to sensory hair cells in the inner ear. Several mechanisms are involved in this process. It seems that aminoglycosides interfere with calcium-receptor–dependent plasma membrane transport channels on hair cells by competitively inhibiting the calcium from binding to these receptors.[34] Furthermore, studies have shown that aminoglycosides irreversibly enter hair cells through one-way channels in the cell membrane, resulting in an accumulation of aminoglycosides within the hair cell.[35] Aminoglycosides interfere with the action of secondary cell messengers within the hair cells and the integrity of the hair cell plasma membrane.[36] Free radicals are believed to be involved in this process, and recent studies have investigated the role of free radical scavengers in preventing gentamicin ototoxicity.[37] Of the different aminoglycosides, streptomycin and gentamicin are predominantly toxic to the vestibular labyrinth (as opposed to cochlea) and hence are most suitable to be used in the treatment of MD. Various techniques have been used to administer aminoglycosides to the inner ear. Systemic administration, transtympanic injection, and the placement of gelfoam soaked in aminoglycoside into the round window niche have all been performed.[38] Shea and Norris[39,40] introduced streptomycin to the inner ear through a fenestration in the lateral semicircular canal. Other novel techniques to deliver aminoglycosides to the inner ear include microcatheters and the Silverstein ear wick.[38]

In general, treatment protocols for aminoglycoside administration can be divided into fixed-dose protocols and titration protocols. Fixed-dose protocols involve the administration of a set dose of aminoglycoside over a predetermined period. The treatment is stopped early only if the patient develops signs of ototoxicity. Titration protocols, on the other hand, aim to administer the drug until the patient begins to show ototoxicity.

Systemic use of streptomycin was first described by Fowler in 1948.[41] Since that time several investigators have published their experience in this area. In 1980, Schuknecht reported on a series of 20 patients treated with 1 g of streptomycin via intramuscular injection every 12 hours.[42] Treatment was continued until there was no response to ice-water calorics in the effected ear. The dose of streptomycin was increased if there was no observed effect after 1 week. Nineteen of the 20 patients had complete relief of vertigo and no patient experienced hearing loss. Although effective in controlling vertigo, this regimen was complicated by patients experiencing severe ataxia during treatment and persisting oscillopsia. This result led others to modify this regimen so that treatment was stopped when the patient began to experience signs of ataxia or oscillopsia. Several investigators using a variation of this method have found intramuscular streptomycin to be effective in controlling vertigo, with no negative effect on hearing or even with improvement in hearing levels.[43-45] Graham and colleagues[46-48] are the exception in this regard, finding that a significant number of their patients suffered hearing loss, with 1 patient experiencing a profound bilateral loss. However, this report is the exception, and common clinical consensus is that intramuscular streptomycin carries little or no risk to hearing. As a result, intramuscular streptomycin using a titration protocol is often recommended for the treatment of symptomatic patients with bilateral MD or MD in a single hearing ear.

Transtympanic administration of aminoglycosides avoids the major drawback of the systemic treatment regiments outlined earlier, namely the oscillopsia that can result from bilateral vestibular hypofunction as well as the risk of nephrotoxicity. Initial studies of transtympanic aminoglycosides used streptomycin.[49] However, animal models have shown that gentamicin is less cochleotoxic than streptomycin when instilled directly into the middle ear, and as a result many investigators have adopted its use.[50] As mentioned earlier, treatment regiments can be broadly divided into fixed-dose protocols and titration protocols.

Although many papers exist related to gentamicin treatment of MD, many of these papers fail to report results according to the AAO-HNS guidelines.[51,52] Kaasinen and colleagues[53] were one of the first groups to publish a large series in which the AAO-HNS guidelines were followed. A total of 93 patients treated with transtympanic gentamicin for MD were followed for 2 years. Gentamicin was administered through a series of transtympanic injections. Rotatory vertigo was abolished in 81% of patients treated. Ten patients suffered dead ears as a response to treatment, and the mean pure tone average decreased by 8.8 dB. Harner and colleagues[54] also published their results from a large series in which the AAO-HNS guidelines were followed. A total of 56 patients were treated with a single transtympanic injection, which was then supplemented by subsequent injections if vertigo control was unsatisfactory; 33 patients had only one injection, 14 patients had 2 injections, 5 patients had 3 injections, and 4 patients received 4 injections. Satisfactory vertigo control was achieved in 82% of patients at 2 years. Hearing results were varied, with some patients showing significant improvement following injection, whereas others experienced a decrease in hearing. The average change in hearing overall was a decrease in the pure tone average of 2.5 dB. Perez and colleagues[55] reported on their experience using repeated transtympanic injections of gentamicin for the treatment of 71 patients with intractable MD. Appropriate diagnostic and reporting guidelines were used. Injections were administered weekly until clinical evidence of vestibular hypofunction became apparent or hearing deteriorated. The round window niche was examined using an endoscope via a myringotomy before treatment to ensure no adhesions were present that might interfere with satisfactory uptake of the gentamicin. Similar results were obtained to the previous studies, with vertigo control rates of approximately 83%. A total of 32% of patients suffered a clinically significant hearing loss as a result of treatment. Using a similar gentamicin protocol, Wu and Minor[56] reported on their experience treating 34 patients with a follow-up period of at least 2 years. A total of 90% of patients experienced excellent vertigo control, with one patient experiencing a severe to profound hearing loss as a result of treatment.

To help draw together these and other results, Cohen-Kerem and colleagues[57] undertook a meta-analysis that combined the results of 15 trials in which the

AAO-HNS guidelines for reporting treatment results in MD were used. This analysis represented 627 patients. Class A vertigo control was achieved in 74.7% of patients and class B control in 92.7% of patients.

This research has led to widespread acceptance of the role of transtympanic gentamicin in treating MD that is refractory to first-line treatments. Much of the ongoing controversy about gentamicin treatment has centered on how various treatment protocols compare with each other and whether a titration protocol results in more patients achieving vertigo control without suffering hearing loss. Cohen-Kerem and colleagues[57] meta-analysis examined this issue. In articles reporting results from patients treated with a fixed-dose protocol, the overall success rate was 68.7% for class A vertigo control and 94.8% for class B control. In articles reporting results from patients treated with a titration protocol, the overall success rate was 75.2% for class A vertigo control and 91.9% for class B control. When the confidence intervals were taken into account, no significant benefit from a titration protocol was identified with regard to vertigo control. Hearing results were similarly compared. Hearing for those treated with fixed-dose protocols was reduced by an average of 5.4 dB, whereas hearing for those treated with a titration protocol was reduced by an average of 0.02 dB. The difference between these results is clinically unimportant, and in addition, when confidence intervals are again considered, they are not statistically significant.

The senior author has used a consistent fixed-dose protocol for treatment of patients with MD since 1988. In several progressive studies the results from this protocol have been published. All results are reported according to the AAO-HNS guidelines for reporting treatment results in MD.[51,52] According to this protocol, gentamicin 40 mg/mL is buffered with sodium bicarbonate to a pH 6.4, giving a final concentration of 26.7 mg/mL. A T-tube grommet is placed in the posteroinferior quadrant of the tympanic membrane, close to the round window, under local anesthetic. Before insertion, the T-tube has a microcatheter attached. One milliliter of the gentamicin solution is administered down the microcatheter with each application. The microcatheter is aspirated before each use. The volume of the microcatheter is 0.35 ml, so effectively, with each administration, 0.65 ml is administered. The treatment is performed in an outpatient setting. Three injections are given each day (7 AM, 1 PM, and 7 PM) for 4 days. The midday injection is given by a physician, whereas a family member is instructed on the technique for the other two. The patient has daily clinical assessment. The patient lies supine with the treated ear upwards for 30 minutes following the injection. The treatment is stopped if the patient develops vertigo, nystagmus, or a deterioration in their audiogram. Vertigo does not usually occur until 2 to 3 days after completion of the treatment. Early in the series, patients were given daily audiologic assessment, but now this is performed at the completion of the treatment. All patients have balance function tests performed before and after the treatment. Comparison of the caloric response between the two is used to measure effectiveness.

In the initial review of this protocol involving 30 patients, 83% of patients treated achieved complete control (vertigo class A) and 17% achieved substantial control (vertigo class B). Ice-water caloric responses were abolished in 53% of patients. Hearing decreased in 27% of patients, and 13% of patients developed a profound hearing loss.[58] A larger series consisting of 90 patients, using the same treatment regimen, was published in 1996.[50] A total of 85% of patients reported complete vertigo control and 9% reported substantial vertigo control. Hearing loss occurred in 23% of patients; 16% of patients suffered a severe to profound hearing loss. The most recent study, in which the minimum follow-up time after treatment was 5 years and the average follow-up time was 15.5 years, again showed consistently good vertigo control.[59]

SUMMARY

Despite many years of research, the exact cause of MD remains elusive. Medical management is the mainstay of treatment of MD. Further research is required to evaluate the effectiveness of many of these treatments. Chemical labyrinthectomy using aminoglycosides is an effective alternative to second-line surgical treatments for those patients in whom medical management is unsuccessful. This article outlines the senior author's protocol for administration of dentamicin for MD and the rationale for this treatment.

REFERENCES

1. Kramer G. Traite des maladies de l'oreille (translated by P Meniere). Paris: Bailliere; 1848.
2. Torok N. Old and new in Meniere disease. Laryngoscope 1977;87:1870–7.
3. Coelho DH, Lalwani AK. Medical management of Menieres disease. Laryngoscope 2008;118:1099–108.
4. Thai-Van H, Bounaix MJ, Fraysse B. Menière's disease: pathophysiology and treatment. Drugs 2001;61:1089–102.
5. Furstenberg AC, Lashmet FH, Lathrop FD. Menieres symptom complex: medical treatment. Ann Otol Rhinol Laryngol 1934;43:1035–47.
6. Thirlwall A, Kundu S. Diuretics for Ménière's disease or syndrome. Cochrane Database Syst Rev 2006;3:CD00359910. DOI:1002/14651858.CD003599.pub2.
7. Dziadziola JK, Laurikainen EL, Rachel JD, et al. Betahistine increases vestibular blood flow. Otolaryngol Head Neck Surg 1999;120:400–5.
8. Botta L, Mira E, Valli S, et al. Effects of betahistine on vestibular receptors of the frog. Acta Otolaryngol 1998;118:519–23.
9. Botta L, Mira E, Valli S, et al. Effects of betahistine metabolites on frog ampullar receptors. Acta Otolaryngol 2000;120:25–7.
10. Arrang JM, Garbarg M, Quach TT, et al. Actions of betahistine at histamine receptors in the brain. Eur J Pharmacol 1985;111:73–84.
11. Frew IJC, Menon GN. Betahistine hydrochloride in Menieres disease. Postgrad Med J 1976;52:501–3.
12. Wilmot TJ, Menon GN. Betahistine in Menieres disease. J Laryngol Otol 1976;90: 833–40.
13. Mira E, Guidetti G, Ghilardi L, et al. Betahistine dihydrochloride in the treatment of peripheral vestibular vertigo. Eur Arch Otorhinolaryngol 2003;260:73–7.
14. Schmidt JT, Huizing EH. The clinical drug trial in Menieres disease with emphasis on the effect of betahistine SR. Acta Otolaryngol Suppl 1992;497:1–189.
15. James A, Burton MJ. Betahistine for Menieres disease or syndrome. Cochrane Database Syst Rev 2001;1:CD001873. DOI:10.1002/14651858.CD001873.
16. Pondugula SR, Sanneman JD, Wangemann P, et al. Glucocorticoids stimulate cation absorption by semicircular canal duct epithelium via epithelial sodium channel. Am J Physiol Renal Physiol 2004;286(6):F1127–35.
17. Trune DR, Kempton JB, Kessi M. Aldosterone (mineralocorticoid) equivalent to prednisolone (glucocorticoid) in reversing hearing loss in MRL/MpJ-Fas1pr autoimmune mice. Laryngoscope 2000;110:1902–6.
18. Itoh A, Sakata E. Treatment of vestibular disorders. Acta Otolaryngol Suppl 1991; 481:617–23.

19. Shea JJ, Ge X. Dexamethasone perfusion of the labyrinth plus intravenous dexamethasone for Menieres disease. Otolaryngol Clin North Am 1996;29:353–9.
20. Silverstein H, Isaacson JE, Olds MJ, et al. Dexamethasone inner ear perfusion for the treatment of Menieres disease: a prospective, randomized, double-blind, crossover trial. Am J Otol 1998;19:196–201.
21. Garduno-Anaya MA, De Toledo HC, Hinojosa-Gonzalez R, et al. Dexamethasone inner ear perfusion by intratympanic injection in unilateral Menieres disease: a two year prospective placebo controlled, double blind, randomized trial. Otolaryngol Head Neck Surg 2005;133:285–94.
22. Boleas-Aguirre MS, Lin FR, Della Santina CC, et al. Longitudinal results with intratympanic dexamethasone in the treatment of Meniere's disease. Otol Neurotol 2008;29(1):33–8.
23. Andrews JC, Ator GA, Honrubia V. The exacerbation of symptoms in Meniere's disease during the premenstrual period. Arch Otolaryngol Head Neck Surg 1992;118:74–8.
24. Price TM, Allen TC, Bowyer DL, et al. Ablation of luteal phase symptoms of Menieres disease with leuprolide. Arch Otolaryngol Head Neck Surg 1994;120:209–11.
25. Gates GA. Innovar treatment for Meniere's disease. Acta Otolaryngol 1999;119(2):189–93.
26. Fattori B, De Iaco G, Vannucci G, et al. Alternobaric and hyperbaric oxygen therapy in the immediate and long term treatment of Menieres disease. Audiology 1996;35:322–34.
27. Yardley L, Kirby S. Evaluation of booklet-based self-management of symptoms in Meniere disease: a randomized controlled trial. Psychosom Med 2006;68:762–9.
28. Mcneill C, Mcmahon CM, Newall P, et al. Hearing aids for Meniere's syndrome: implications of hearing fluctuation. J Am Acad Audiol 2008;19:430–4.
29. Gates GA, Verrall A, Green JD, et al. Meniett clinical trial: long-term follow-up. Arch Otolaryngol Head Neck Surg 2006;132:1311–6.
30. Mattox DE, Reichert M. Meniett device for Menieres disease: use and compliance at 3 to 5 years. Otol Neurotol 2007;29:29–32.
31. Dornhoffer JL, King D. The effect of the Meniett device in patients with Menieres disease: long-term results. Otol Neurotol 2008;28:868–74.
32. Rajan GP, Din S, Atlas MD. Longterm effects of the Meniett device in Menieres disease: the Western Australian experience. J Laryngol Otol 2005;119:391–5.
33. Thomsen J, Sass K, Odkvist L, et al. Local overpressure treatment reduces vestibular symptoms in patients with Menieres disease: a clinical, randomized, multicenter, double-blind placebo-controlled study. Otol Neurotol 2005;26:68–73.
34. Ohmori H. Mechano-electrical transduction currents in isolated vestibular hair cells of the chick. J Physiol 1985;359:189–217.
35. Waguespack J, Ricci A. Aminoglycoside ototoxicity: permeant drugs cause permanent hair cell loss. J Physiol 2005;567:359–60.
36. Williams S, Zenner H, Schacht J. Three molecular steps of aminoglycoside ototoxicity demonstrated in outer hair cells. Hear Res 1987;30:11–8.
37. Sha SH, Qiu JH, Schacht J. Aspirin to prevent gentamicin induced hearing loss. N Engl J Med 2006;354:1856–7.
38. Hoffmann KK, Silverstein H. Inner ear perfusion: indications and applications. Curr Opin Otolaryngol Head Neck Surg 2003;11(5):334–9.
39. Shea JJ. Perfusion of the inner ear with streptomycin. Am J Otol 1989;10:150–5.
40. Shea JJ, Norris CH. Streptomycin perfusion of the labyrinth. In: Nadol JB, editor. Menieres disease. Proceedings of the Second International Symposium on

Menieres disease, June 20–22, 1988. Cambridge (MA): Kugler and Khedini Publ; 1989.

41. Fowler EP. Streptomycin treatment for vertigo. Trans Am Acad Ophthalmol Otolaryngol 1948;52:293–301.

42. Wilson RW, Schuknecht HF. Update on the use of streptomycin therapy for Menieres disease. Am J Otol 1980;2:108–11.

43. Schuknecht HF. Ablation therapy for the relief of Menieres disease. Laryngoscope 1956;66:859–70.

44. Khetarpal U, Schuknecht HF. Temporal bone findings in a case of bilateral Menieres disease treated by parenteral streptomycin and endolymphatic shunt. Laryngoscope 1990;100:407–14.

45. Silverstein H. Streptomycin treatment for Menieres disease. Ann Otol Rhinol Laryngol Suppl 1984;112:44–8.

46. Graham MD, Sataloff RT, Kemink JL. Titration streptomycin therapy for bilateral Menieres disease: a preliminary report. Otolaryngol Head Neck Surg 1984;92: 440–7.

47. Larouere MJ, Zappia JJ, Graham MD. Titration streptomycin therapy in Menieres disease: current concepts. Am J Otol 1993;14(5):474–7.

48. Langman AW, Kemink JL, Graham MD. Titration streptomycin therapy for bilateral Menieres disease: follow up report. Ann Otol Rhinol Laryngol 1990;99:923–6.

49. Schuknecht H. Ablation therapy in the management of Menieres disease. Acta Otolaryngol Suppl 1957;132:1–42.

50. Commins DJ, Nedzelski JM. Topical drugs in the treatment of Menieres disease. Curr Opin Otolaryngol Head Neck Surg 1996;4:319–23.

51. Subcommittee on Equilibrium. Menieres disease: criteria for diagnosis and evaluation of therapy for reporting. AAO-HNS Bull 1985;7:6–7.

52. Committee on Hearing and Equilibrium. Committee on Hearing and Equilibrium guidelines for the diagnosis and evaluation of therapy in Menieres Disease. Otolaryngol Head Neck Surg 1995;113:181–5.

53. Kaasinen S, Pyykko I, Ishizaki H, et al. Intratympanic gentamicin in Menieres disease. Acta Otolaryngol (Stockh) Suppl 1998;118:294–8.

54. Harner SG, Driscoll CL, Facer W, et al. Long-term follow-up of transtympanic gentamicin for Menieres syndrome. Otol Neurotol 2001;22:210–4.

55. Perez N, Martin E, Garcia-Tapia R. Intratympanic gentamicin for intractable Menieres disease. Laryngoscope 2003;113:456–64.

56. Wu IC, Minor LB. Longterm hearing outcome in patients receiving intratympanic gentamicin for Menieres disease. Laryngoscope 2003;113:815–20.

57. Cohen-Kerem R, Kisilevsky V, Einarson TR, et al. Intratympanic gentamicin for Menieres disease: a meta-analysis. Laryngoscope 2004;114:2085–91.

58. Nedzelski JM, Schessel D, Bryce G, et al. Chemical labyrinthectomy: local application for the treatment of unilateral Menieres disease. Am J Otol 1992;13:18–22.

59. Bodmer D, Morong S, Stewart C, et al. Long-term vertigo control in patients after intratympanic gentamicin instillation for Menieres Disease. Otol Neurotol 2007;28: 1140–4.

Endolymphatic Sac Shunt, Labyrinthectomy, and Vestibular Nerve Section in Meniere's Disease

Karen B. Teufert, MD[a],*, Joni Doherty, MD, PhD[b]

KEYWORDS

- Surgical treatment of vertigo • Vertigo • Imbalance
- Meniere's disease • Endolymphatic sac shunt
- Vestibular nerve section • Labyrinthectomy

Surgery has long been used to control disabling vertigo of Meniere's disease and other peripheral vestibular disorders refractory to medical measures, with each surgical procedure having many technical variations.

The history of vestibular nerve section (VNS) was recently reviewed.[1] It was first attempted in 1898, with microscopic technique later introduced by William House in 1960. The retrolabyrinthine and retrosigmoid-internal auditory canal (IAC) approaches for VNS were popularized in the 1980s.[2–4] Transmastoid labyrinthectomy, the gold standard surgical technique for complete removal of all neuroepithelial elements of the ear causing disabling disequilibrium, was described as early as1904.[5–8] When properly performed, transmastoid labyrinthectomy eliminates all vestibular function in the diseased periphery, but at the expense of any remaining cochlear function. Another common treatment option for patients with intractable Meniere's disease, endolymphatic sac (ES) surgery, has stood the test of time for 75 years.[9] House[10] described and popularized endolymphatic sac surgery (the shunt procedure) in the early 1960s.

For patients with unilateral disease, the procedures of choice are endolymphatic mastoid shunt (**Figs. 1** and **2**) and vestibular nerve section (translabyrinthine, retrolabyrinthine, retrosigmoid and middle cranial fossa VNS) (**Fig. 3**). These procedures are

[a] House Ear Institute, Los Angeles, CA, USA
[b] Division of Otolaryngology/Head and Neck Surgery, University of California San Diego, San Diego, CA, USA
* Corresponding author.
E-mail address: KTeufert@hei.org

Otolaryngol Clin N Am 43 (2010) 1091–1111
doi:10.1016/j.otc.2010.05.014
0030-6665/10/$ – see front matter

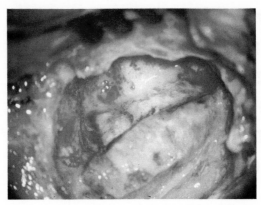

Fig. 1. Endolymphatic sac surgery: the sigmoid sinus and dura are decompressed and the endolymphatic sac is identified. (*Courtesy of* Antonio De la Cruz, MD, House Ear Clinic, Los Angeles, CA.)

preferred over labyrinthectomy (**Fig. 4**) because cochlear nerve integrity is preserved, leaving open the possibility of future cochlear implantation should bilateral profound hearing loss develop.

Telischi and Luxford[11] published statistically valid long-term results in endolymphatic sac surgery. This procedure is recommended as the surgical procedure of first choice. Sixty-three percent of patients undergoing sac surgery do not require further surgical procedures and an additional 17% have only revisions of the endolymphatic sac shunt. Thus, 80% never require a destructive procedure and 93% report no further dizziness or mild to no disability 13.5 years later. The sac procedure has only a 2% risk of hearing loss or hearing worsening. Patients who fail sac procedures, or who are severely symptomatic, show a 90% vertigo cure rate to vestibular neurectomy.

SURGICAL MANAGEMENT

Several procedures are available for the surgical treatment of Meniere's disease. The surgeon should take into consideration severity of disease, hearing status, and presence of unilateral versus bilateral disease when selecting an approach.

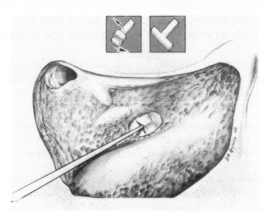

Fig. 2. Endolymphatic sac surgery: The endolymphatic sac is incised and a T-strut is placed in the sac. (*Courtesy of* House Ear Institute, Los Angeles, CA; with permission.)

MASTOIDECTOMY

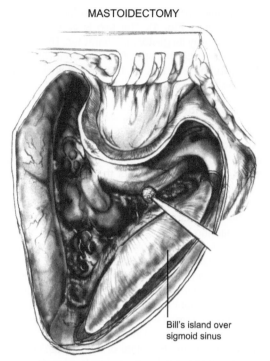

Bill's island over
sigmoid sinus

Fig. 3. Mastoidectomy with exposure of the sigmoid sinus. Note that a small bony island is left over the sinus to protect it from the shaft of the bur. (*From* House JW, Friedman RA. Translabyrinthine approach. In: Brackmann DE, Shelton C, Arriaga MA, editors. Otologic surgery. 2nd edition. Philadelphia: WB Saunders; 2001. p. 511–19; with permission.)

Endolymphatic drainage procedures can be divided into external shunts that attempt to drain excessive endolymph from the endolymphatic sac into the mastoid or subarachnoid space (ie, endolymphatic sac shunt) and internal shunts that attempt to drain excessive endolymph into the perilymphatic space (ie, cochleosacculotomy [labyrinthotomy]).

Approaches that transverse the labyrinth, such as labyrinthectomy and translabyrinthine vestibular neurectomy, sacrifice hearing and are useful in patients without useful hearing. Posterior approaches that spare the labyrinth (retrolabyrinthine and retrosigmoid vestibular neurectomy) provide varying degrees of cerebellopontine angle (CPA) exposure with an opportunity for hearing preservation. Superior approaches permit unroofing of the IAC and an opportunity for hearing preservation, such as middle fossa vestibular neurectomy; however, this procedure has fallen out of favor because of increased risk for facial nerve injury or transient palsy, compared with the other approaches.

Endolymphatic Sac Shunt

A postauricular incision is made approximately 2 cm posterior to the sulcus, and the mastoid cortex is cleaned of periosteal soft tissues. A routine mastoidectomy is performed and then extended to include dissection to at least 1 cm posterior to the sigmoid sinus. Additional bone removal is done so that the dura of the posterior fossa is skeletonized from the sigmoid sinus posteriorly to the posterior semicircular canal anteriorly and the endolymphatic sac inferiorly. Exposure of the posterior fossa dura is extended toward the jugular bulb and into the retrofacial air cells, allowing a large decompression of the sac (see **Fig. 1**). The sac is carefully entered with a sharp hook and the lumen identified by its glistening character. The lumen is widely opened with a long, blunt, right-angle hook with specific attention toward the duct. A T-shaped silastic is placed into the lumen (see **Fig. 2**). The wound is closed by use of subcutaneous absorbable sutures followed by skin sutures.

Cochleosacculotomy (Labyrinthotomy)

Cochleosacculotomy is performed under local anesthesia and is the procedure of choice for patients who, for health reasons, are at risk from the stress of postoperative vertigo and who should not have general anesthesia, as well as for elderly patients who often compensate poorly to procedures that ablate vestibular function. It has the advantage of being technically simple to perform, is almost totally free of morbidity, and carries little or no risk of mortality. However, it results in sensorineural hearing loss, and is therefore usually used in patients with preexisting severe-to-profound sensorineural hearing loss.

The cochleosacculotomy operation consists of creating a fracture disruption by impaling the osseous spiral lamina and cochlear duct with a pick introduced through the round window. Usually, the round window niche accommodates a 3-mm right-angle pick without removal of bone. The pick is advanced through the round window membrane, which may or may not be visible. The pick is guided in the direction of the oval window while hugging the lateral wall of the inner ear to ensure that the cochlear duct is traversed. When the pick has been introduced to its full 3-mm length, the end of the pick will be located beneath the footplate of the stapes. Occasionally, the subiculum, which is a ridge of bone lying in the boundary between the round window niche and sinus tympani, interferes with introduction of the pick. It can readily be shaved down with a 2-mm burr. Occasionally, the overhanging bony lip of the round window niche must be removed to accommodate the pick. In this case, a 2-mm (rather than a 3-mm) pick is used to avoid excessively deep penetration into the vestibule and possible injury to the utricular macula. Rarely, a high jugular bulb blocks access to the round window niche, in which case it may be necessary to abort the operation.

The pick is withdrawn and the perforation in the round window membrane is sealed by a tissue graft of perichondrium or adipose tissue. The operation is terminated by returning the tympanomeatal flap to its original position. A piece of Gelfoam is placed in the canal to maintain slight pressure on the skin flap. Cotton is placed in the ear canal.

Labyrinthectomy

An incision is made approximately 1 cm above and behind the postauricular crease and follows the contour of the auricle. A plane is established in the galea aponeurotic layer lateral to the temporalis muscle and the auricle is turned forward. A thick periosteal flap is created by incising this tissue along the linear temporalis just anterior to the incision line and then inferior to the mastoid tip. This flap is elevated off the mastoid cortex and retracted forward with a large self-retaining retractor. The staggered two-layer incision provides better closure to prevent cerebrospinal fluid leaks.

The high-speed drill with a large cutting burr and constant suction irrigation is used to perform a cortical mastoidectomy. The posterior external bony canal wall is thinned, the bone over the tegmen is thinned, and the sigmoid sinus is skeletonized. The bone over the sinus is frequently eggshelled and decompressed by collapsing it with thumb pressure, leaving tiny, fragmented pieces of bone over the highly vulnerable sigmoid sinus to protect it from damage from instruments entering and exiting the wound (see **Fig. 3**). The sinus is easily collapsed and gives needed exposure medially. The sinodural angle is opened as far back on the cortex as possible. Because the vestibule lies under the facial nerve anteriorly, an angulated view via the sinodural angle is necessary to visualize the contents of the vestibule and eventually identify landmarks used to excise the superior vestibular nerve.

Bone over the posterior fossa dura is thinned out but not removed. The labyrinth is skeletonized and the cells of the mastoid tip are opened. The labyrinthectomy is performed by opening the crown of the lateral (horizontal) semicircular canal on its posterior border and following the half-opened canal posteriorly to the posterior canal. The lateral canal is only half opened to protect the external genu of the facial nerve until careful trimming can be done. The posterior canal, having been opened, can be traced to its confluence with the superior semicircular canal, where the two canals combine to become the common crus (see **Fig. 4**). The common crus may then be followed directly forward to the vestibule (**Fig. 5**).

The posterior surface of the facial nerve over the external genu is now thinned carefully, and the anterior limb of the posterior canal is followed to its ampulla at the inferior pole of the elliptical recess. The lateral canal is opened anteriorly and medially to its ampullated end, and the ampulla of the superior canal identified next to that of the lateral is opened. The superior canal is opened along the tegmen throughout its course, which curves back to the common crus.

With all the canals and the vestibule opened, all soft-tissue elements of the membranous labyrinth should be removed. This step would be the normal end point of the postauricular, postganglionic labyrinthectomy but only sets the stage to skeletonize the IAC in a translabyrinthine vestibular nerve section and preganglionic denervation (**Fig. 6**).

Translabyrinthine Vestibular Neurectomy

A mastoidectomy and labyrinthectomy are performed as previously described under labyrinthectomy. A key factor in successful exploration of the IAC is clear identification

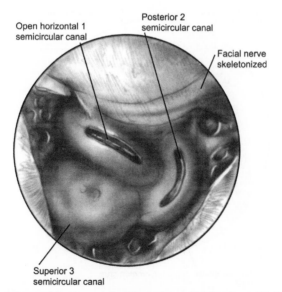

Open horizontal 1 semicircular canal

Posterior 2 semicircular canal

Facial nerve skeletonized

Superior 3 semicircular canal

Fig. 4. Opening of the semicircular canals. (*From* House JW, Friedman RA. Translabyrinthine approach. In: Brackmann DE, Shelton C, Arriaga MA, editors. Otologic surgery. 2nd edition. Philadelphia: WB Saunders; 2001. p. 511–19; with permission.)

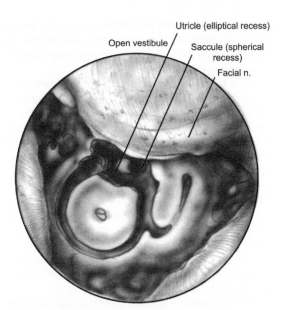

Utricle (elliptical recess)

Open vestibule

Saccule (spherical recess)

Facial n.

Fig. 5. Opening of the vestibule. (*From* House JW, Friedman RA. Translabyrinthine approach. In: Brackmann DE, Shelton C, Arriaga MA, editors. Otologic surgery. 2nd edition. Philadelphia: WB Saunders; 2001. p. 511–19; with permission.)

of the IAC contents. Identification is possible only if the soft-tissue contents are not violated in the removal of bone during IAC skeletonization. Loss of part or all of any of the soft-tissue landmarks places all the other contents at great risk because of the difficulty in differentiating the nerves from one another. The purpose in using the

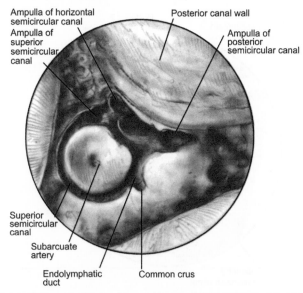

Ampulla of horizontal semicircular canal

Ampulla of superior semicircular canal

Posterior canal wall

Ampulla of posterior semicircular canal

Superior semicircular canal

Subarcuate artery

Endolymphatic duct

Common crus

Fig. 6. Cleaning of the vestibule. (*From* House JW, Friedman RA. Translabyrinthine approach. In: Brackmann DE, Shelton C, Arriaga MA, editors. Otologic surgery. 2nd edition. Philadelphia: WB Saunders; 2001. p. 511–19; with permission.)

facial nerve-vestibular nerve tissue plane when dissecting the IAC is to enable identi-fication of the facial nerve in its normal position and extend the dissection into the diseased area, where those relationships are sometimes more difficult to ascertain.

A useful technique for IAC skeletonization is blue lining the IAC throughout the area to be opened. The thin bony cover protects the soft-tissue structures within the IAC. Blue lining actually starts at the vestibule because this is where the bone is the thin-nest. The nerves of the IAC exit into the bony labyrinth through perforations in the thin bone separating the fundus of the IAC from the vestibule. This naturally blue-lined area can be used as a starting point for skeletonization of the remainder of the canal. Removal of bone should extend to the porus acusticus and should cover 180° of the lateral side of the canal. The general orientation of the IAC is that the fundus is lateral just medial to the vestibule. The superior border is along a line drawn between the superior semicircular canal ampulla and the sinodural angle, and the inferior border is along the line starting at the posterior semicircular canal ampulla drawn posteriorly parallel to the superior border. The IAC angles away from the surgeon in an anterolateral-to-posteromedial direction deep to the sigmoid sinus (**Fig. 7**).

Once the IAC is adequately skeletonized, the thin bone over the canal is lifted away with a small right-angle pick. The perforated area where the superior vestibular nerve enters both the lateral and the superior ampullae is thinned carefully, and a 1-mm hook is used to avulse the superior vestibular nerve from the vestibular nerve recess that it makes in the labyrinthine bone lateral to the fallopian canal. As the superior vestibular nerve is reflected, the facial nerve comes into view deep to the plane of dissection (**Fig. 8**). If the facial nerve is not immediately visible, the hook can be used to palpate the bone of the vestibular nerve recess (Bill's bar, or the lateral wall of the fallopian canal) until the edge of the fallopian canal is found and the hook is easily inserted into this labyrinthine segment of the canal.

With the superior vestibular nerve separated from the facial nerve, the inferior vestibular nerve is also avulsed with the singular nerve to the posterior semicircular canal. Because the singular nerve frequently leaves the inferior nerve midway out of

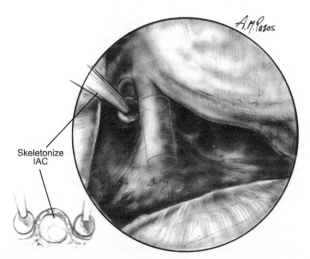

Fig. 7. Skeletonization of the internal auditory canal (IAC). (*From* House JW, Friedman RA. Translabyrinthine approach. In: Brackmann DE, Shelton C, Arriaga MA, editors. Otologic surgery. 2nd edition. Philadelphia: WB Saunders; 2001. p. 511–19; with permission.)

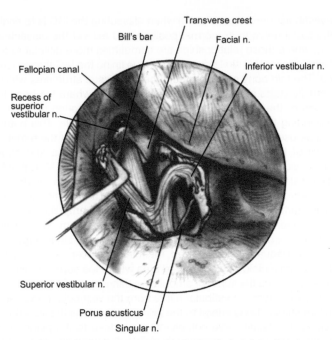

Transverse crest

Bill's bar

Facial n.

Inferior vestibular n.

Fallopian canal

Recess of
superior
vestibular n.

Superior vestibular n.

Porus acusticus

Singular n.

Fig. 8. The superior vestibular nerve is avulsed and reflected and the facial nerve is visualized. (*From* House JW, Friedman RA. Translabyrinthine approach. In: Brackmann DE, Shelton C, Arriaga MA, editors. Otologic surgery, 2nd edition. Philadelphia: WB Saunders; 2001. p. 511–19; with permission.)

the IAC, the surgeon must be careful to check for it. Failure to include the singular nerve may cause failure of the operation.

Scarpa's ganglion lies midway out of the IAC. The avulsed ends of the two vestibular nerves are reflected and the fused nerves sectioned medial to the ganglion. The specimen is sent to a pathologist for examination (**Fig. 9**).

Although the cochlear nerve may also be sectioned, this action would preclude its use in a cochlear implant if that opportunity arises. Generally, implantation is not a strong consideration, but sometimes a cochlear nerve section may be entertained as a possible solution to overwhelming tinnitus symptoms. Because elimination of tinnitus is not guaranteed, this approach is rarely encouraged.

Hemostasis is achieved through bipolar cautery and the application of bovine collagen. Control of cerebrospinal fluid leak is achieved through dural closure with 4-0 silk sutures when possible, but primarily through packing. The IAC and labyrinthine defects are sealed with strips of adipose tissue obtained from the abdominal wall, and the mastoid incision is closed with interrupted, slow-absorbing sutures in a 2-layer fashion: first, the thick periosteal flap and then a subcuticular closure of the skin. Steri-Strips (3M St Paul, MN, USA) are placed over the incision and a mastoid dressing is applied.

Retrolabyrinthine Vestibular Neurectomy

Following a complete mastoidectomy, bone around the superior and posterior semicircular canals is removed to skeletonize the posterior fossa dura anterior to the sigmoid sinus. This procedure is paramount for adequate exposure of the approach. Exposure of the posterior fossa dura behind the sigmoid sinus is necessary to permit

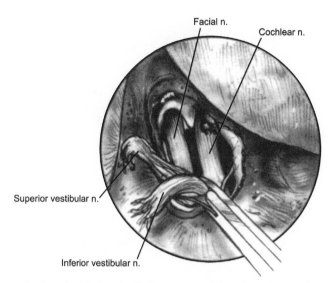

Fig. 9. The avulsed ends of the vestibular nerves are reflected and the fused nerves sectioned medial to Scarpa's ganglion. (*From* House JW, Friedman RA. Translabyrinthine approach. In: Brackmann DE, Shelton C, Arriaga MA, editors. Otologic surgery. 2nd edition. Philadelphia: WB Saunders; 2001. p. 511–19; with permission.)

extradural compression of the sinus for adequate CPA exposure (**Fig. 10A**). An anterior-based U-shaped incision is made in the dura from superior to inferior, taking care to preserve the endolymphatic sac with the apex of the incision just medial to the sigmoid sinus (see **Fig. 10B**). The dura is reflected anteriorly and the intracranial dissection is done to release arachnoid and cerebrospinal fluid. The contents of the cerebellopontine angle are exposed and the seventh and eighth cranial nerves are identified (see **Fig. 10C**). The vestibular division of the eighth nerve is sectioned and seen to retract, suggesting complete section of vestibular fibers (see **Fig. 10D**). The dura is then approximated with a running suture, the cavity is obliterated with abdominal fat, and a titanium mesh cranioplasty is performed.

Although this approach was originally used for trigeminal nerve section in cases of refractory tic douloureux, it is now commonly employed for vestibular neurectomy and microvascular decompression. An advantage of this approach for vestibular neurectomy is that the endolymphatic sac is in the surgical field. In Meniere's disease cases, an extensive endolymphatic sac decompression can be performed at the time of vestibular neurectomy.

Retrosigmoid Vestibular Neurectomy

The retrosigmoid approach for VNS is currently the most commonly used because of its short operative time and ease compared with the other approaches. A posterior fossa craniotomy is performed immediately behind the lateral sinus and the cerebellum is retracted to give exposure to the seventh and eight cranial nerves and the IAC.

The first major landmark seen in the posterior fossa above the jugular foramen is the white linear fold of dura: the jugular dural fold. The dural fold extends approximately 2 cm from the anterior aspect of the foramen magnum, overlying the junction of the lateral sinus and jugular bulb and attaching to the temporal bone 7 mm medial to the endolymphatic duct. The dural fold lies 7 to 9 mm lateral to the exit of the ninth nerve. The anterior aspect of the fold usually points to the eighth cranial nerve, which is 7 to

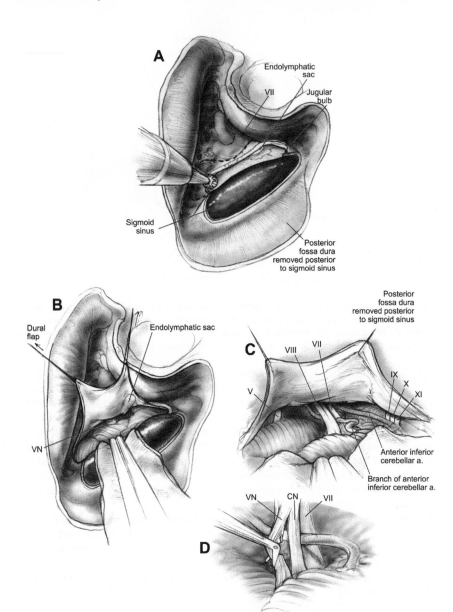

Fig. 10. (*A–D*) The posterior fossa dura as seen through the retrolabyrinthine approach. (*A*) Exposure of the posterior fossa dura. (*B*) Dural incision anterior to the sigmoid sinus. (*C*) Exposure of cranial nerves V, VII, VIII, IX, X, and XI. (*D*) After the cleavage plane is visualized under high-power magnification, a longitudinal incision is made in the cleavage plane, the cochlear and vestibular fibers are separated, and the vestibular nerve (VN) is transected. CN, cochlear nerve. (*From* Silverstein H, Rosenberg SI. Retrolabyrinthine/retrosigmoid vestibular neurectomy. In: Brackmann DE, Shelton C, Arriaga MA, editors. Otologic surgery. 2nd edition. Philadelphia: WE Saunders; 2001. p. 397–406; with permission.)

10 mm medial. Using a diamond drill bit, the posterior wall of the IAC is removed to the singular canal, thereby exposing the branches of the eighth cranial nerve (**Fig. 11**A). The superior vestibular nerve and the singular nerve are sectioned (see **Fig. 11**B). The inferior vestibular fibers that innervate the saccule are not divided because of their close association with cochlear fibers. The saccule has no known vestibular function in humans, so sparing these fibers does not result in postoperative vertigo attacks.

Middle Cranial Fossa Vestibular Neurectomy

An incision is made 1 cm anterior to the tragus and above the zygomatic arch and is extended superiorly in a gently curving fashion (**Fig. 12**). The midportion of the incision curves posteriorly, which keeps it in the hair of most patients with male pattern baldness. An inferiorly based U-shaped flap is fashioned of the temporalis muscle and fascia and is reflected inferiorly.

By use of a cutting burr, a craniotomy opening is made in the squamous portion of the temporal bone. It is located approximately two-thirds anterior and one-third posterior to the external auditory canal and is approximately 5 × 5 cm (**Fig. 13**). Anterior placement of the craniotomy is important for adequate exposure. This bone flap is based on the root of the zygoma as close to the floor of the middle fossa as possible. During creation of this flap, care is taken to avoid laceration of the underlying dura. The bone flap is set aside for later replacement.

The dura is elevated from the floor of the middle fossa and any bone edges are drilled away as close as possible to the floor of the middle fossa. The initial landmark is the middle meningeal artery, which marks the anterior extent of the dissection. Frequently, venous bleeding will be encountered from this area and can be controlled

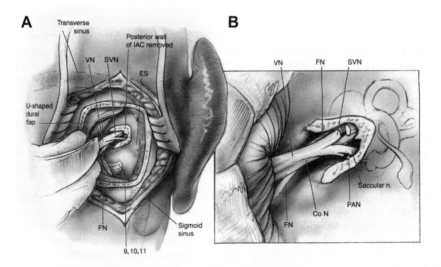

Fig. 11. (A) The posterior wall of the internal auditory canal (IAC) is removed, exposing the branches if the eighth cranial nerve. (B) The superior vestibular nerve (SVN) and posterior ampullary nerves (PAN) are transected while the saccular nerve is spared. This allows for complete denervation of the vestibular labyrinth without damaging the cochlear nerve (Co N). FN, facial nerve; 9, 10, 11, cranial nerves IX, X, XI; VN, vestibular nerve; ES, endolymphatic sac. Retrolabyrinthine/retrosigmoid vestibular neurectomy. (*From* Silverstein H, Rosenberg SI. Retrolabyrinthine/retrosigmoid vestibular neurectomy. In: Brackmann DE, Shelton C, Arriaga MA, editors. Otologic surgery. 2nd edition. Philadelphia: WE Saunders; 2001. p. 397–406; with permission.)

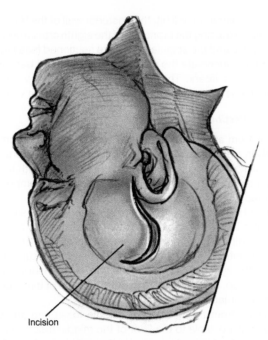

Incision

Fig. 12. Incision begins in the pretragal area and extends 7 to 8 cm superiorly in gently curving fashion. (*From* Shelton C, Brackmann DE, House WF. Middle fossa approach. In: Brackmann DE, Shelton C, Arriaga MA, editors. Otologic surgery. 2nd edition. Philadelphia: WB Saunders; 2001. p. 503–10; with permission.)

with Surgicel (Ethicon Inc, Somerville, NJ, USA). Dissection of the dura proceeds in a posterior-to-anterior manner. In approximately 5% of cases, the geniculate ganglion of the facial nerve will be dehiscent, but injury can be avoided with dural elevation.[12] The petrous ridge is identified and care is taken not to injure the superior petrosal sinus. The arcuate eminence and greater superficial petrosal nerve are identified. These are the major landmarks to the subsequent intratemporal dissection. Once the dura has been elevated, typically with a suction irrigator and a blunt dural elevator, the House-Urban middle fossa retractor is placed to support the temporal lobe. To maintain a secure position, the teeth of the retaining retractor should be locked against the bony margins of the craniotomy window and the tip of the retractor must be placed beneath the petrous ridge (**Fig. 14**).

The greater superficial petrosal nerve is located medial to the middle meningeal artery (**Fig. 15**). Using a large diamond drill and continuous suction irrigation, the superior semicircular canal is identified. Bone is removed at the medial aspect of the petrous ridge at the bisection of the angle formed by the greater superficial petrosal nerve and the superior semicircular canal, as described by Garcia-Ibanez.[13] The IAC is identified in this medial location and traced laterally. The dura of the posterior fossa is widely exposed (2 cm) and the circumference of the porus acusticus is exposed for approximately 240° (**Fig. 16**). As the dissection proceeds laterally, it must narrow to about 90° because of the encroachment of the cochlea and superior semicircular canal. At the lateral end of the IAC, Bill's bar and the labyrinthine facial nerve are exposed.

Once the IAC is unroofed from the fundus to the porus, dura over the superior vestibular nerve is opened with a 1.0-mm hook (**Fig. 17**). The nerve is identified and

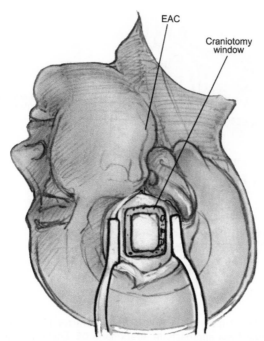

EAC

Craniotomy
window

Fig. 13. Two-thirds of the craniotomy window is located anterior to the external auditory canal (EAC). (*From* Shelton C, Brackmann DE, House WF. Middle fossa approach. In: Brackmann DE, Shelton C, Arriaga MA, editors. Otologic surgery. 2nd edition. Philadelphia: WB Saunders; 2001. p. 503–10; with permission.)

cut sharply with a neurectomy knife distal to the vestibular crest. Avulsion of the superior vestibular nerve with a hook is discouraged because of the high incidence of deafness that can result from either traction or vascular injury to the cochlear nerve.

The meatal dura is incised along the posterior edge towards the porus. The cut end of the superior vestibular nerve is retracted with a microsuction to expose the saccular and singular branches of the inferior vestibular nerve, which are then sectioned with a neurectomy knife. The entire vestibular nerve is stabilized with the suction while the vestibulofacial anastomoses are cut sharply with a neurectomy scissor. The vestibular nerve is now everted with Scarpa's ganglion in full view. The vessels are coagulated and the nerve is then resected proximal to the ganglion with neurectomy scissors (**Fig. 18**). The facial nerve should only be partially exposed, retaining most of its dural cover for protection. The cochlear nerve is hidden beneath the facial nerve and should not be exposed.

Bone wax is applied on the middle fossa floor and abdominal fat is used to close the defect in the IAC. The House-Urban retractor is removed and the temporal lobe is allowed to re-expand. The craniotomy flap is replaced.

The wound is closed with absorbable subcutaneous sutures over a Penrose drain, if indicated. This drain is typically removed on the first postoperative day. A mastoid-type pressure dressing is maintained for 4 days postoperatively.

Although not severe, postoperative pain after the middle fossa approach can be more intense than that from the other approaches. This pain results from muscle spasm from division of the temporalis muscle. Some degree of temporary trismus may also result. Routine postoperative analgesics are usually sufficient to control

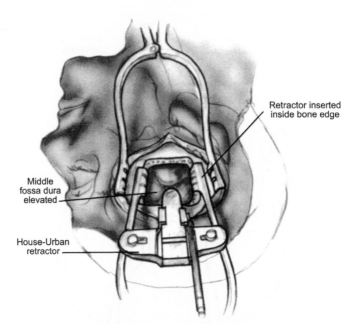

Fig. 14. Temporal lobe is supported by House-Urban retractor. (*From* Shelton C, Brackmann DE, House WF. Middle fossa approach. In: Brackmann DE, Shelton C, Arriaga MA, editors. Otologic surgery. 2nd edition. Philadelphia: WB Saunders; 2001. p. 503–10; with permission.)

this pain. However, combined with a slightly increased incidence of facial palsy post-operatively and the relative technical difficulty compared with other approaches, the middle fossa approach has fallen out of favor for VNS.

SURGICAL OUTCOMES

A series of 3 studies on the surgical treatment of vertigo was recently conducted at the House Ear Institute. In the first study, the primary aim was to describe efficacy of surgical procedures for the treatment of vertigo based on the subjects' perspective about the characteristics of their dizziness symptoms in an attempt to add another dimension to evaluating the difficult topic of outcomes of surgical procedures for vertigo.[14] In addition to reviewing surgical experience with the treatment of vertigo for 3637 procedures performed over a 30-year period, including endolymphatic sac shunt, translabyrinthine, retrolabyrinthine, retrosigmoid and middle cranial fossa vestibular nerve section, and labyrinthectomy, a questionnaire was also sent to a random sample of subjects for each major procedure type to assess frequency, severity, interference, and amount of disability for both vertigo and imbalance before and after surgery, and the postoperative time course of improvements. Questionnaires were completed by 28 subjects with ES shunt, 54 with vestibular nerve section, and 14 with labyrinthectomy.

All 3 of the procedure groups rated their current vertigo characteristics as significantly improved relative to before surgery and both the ES and VNS groups also rated all characteristics of their imbalance as improved (all $P \leq .001$), although the VNS group had a much higher rate of current imbalance. The small group of labyrinthectomy subjects did not rate any of their imbalance characteristics as significantly improved and many rated imbalance as worse after surgery. Glasscock and

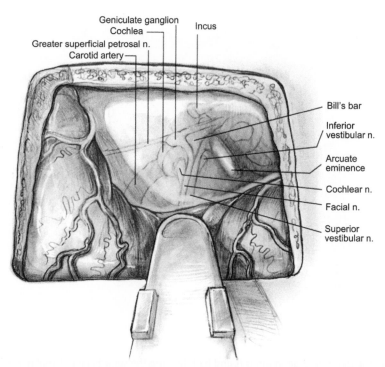

Geniculate ganglion
Cochlea
Incus
Greater superficial petrosal n.
Carotid artery

Bill's bar

Inferior
vestibular n.

Arcuate
eminence

Cochlear n.

Facial n.

Superior
vestibular n.

Fig. 15. The greater superficial petrosal nerve is identified medial to the middle meningeal artery. (*From* Shelton C, Brackmann DE, House WF. Middle fossa approach. In: Brackmann DE, Shelton C, Arriaga MA, editors. Otologic surgery. 2nd edition. Philadelphia: WB Saunders; 2001. p. 503–10; with permission.)

colleagues,[15] Schuknecht,[16] and Kemink and colleagues[17] have all reported similar results. It has been noted in the literature that the elderly may have an increased incidence of postoperative disequilibrium.[17] It was also duly noted in the most recent study that the subjects undergoing labyrinthectomy tended to be a little older on average than those in the other two groups.[11] However, no significant relationship between age at surgery and any of the current dizziness characteristics was found.

The majority of all 3 groups indicated that they still have imbalance, although it may be improved. The authors found no significant differences between groups in any of the current vertigo characteristics or the change in the American Academy of Otolaryngology-Head and Neck Surgery (AAO-HNS) disability rating from before to after surgery. However, frequency, severity, and interference of imbalance did differ between groups, with the ES group having the best ratings and the labyrinthectomy group the poorest. The differences between the ES and VNS groups were also statistically significant. Their ratings of before-surgery dizziness symptoms did not differ, indicating that in this particular subject sample, the two groups had similar severity of disease prior to surgery.

Others have reported recurrent vertigo or constant disequilibrium in subjects following vestibular nerve section.[18,19] Thedinger and Thedinger[18] suggested several possible causes for this, including incomplete nerve section, neuroma formation, unsatisfactory compensation processes, vestibular dysfunction in the contralateral ear, nerve regeneration, and the possibility of nonotologic vertigo. More recently, Moon and Hain[19] reported on 3 patients with delayed return of spinning spells following vestibular

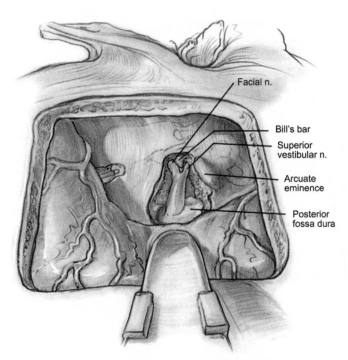

Fig. 16. The geniculate ganglion is found by following the superficial petrosal nerve posteriorly. Bill's bar separates the facial nerve from the superior vestibular nerve at the lateral end of the internal auditory canal. The internal auditory canal is skeletonized through the entire length. Bone is removed around the porus acusticus, uncovering dura of the posterior fossa. (*From* Shelton C, Brackmann DE, House WF. Middle fossa approach. In: Brackmann DE, Shelton C, Arriaga MA, editors. Otologic surgery. 2nd edition. Philadelphia: WB Saunders; 2001. p. 503–10; with permission.)

neurectomy for Meniere's disease. They suggest the cause to be irritable vestibular nerve fibers that may be located in a neuroma, spared by the original operation, or regenerated after surgery. Treatment with agents used for neuralgia proved effective. The question of whether bilateral vestibular dysfunction may contribute to patients' perceptions of continuing spinning dizziness after VNS is unresolved. However, many would argue that once vestibular function is eliminated in one ear, it is theoretically impossible to experience vertigo based on dysfunction on the contralateral side because vertigo is a result of reduced vestibular response of one side relative to the other.

The authors compared labyrinthectomy with and without nerve section. Although all subjects with translabyrinthine vestibular nerve section (TLVNS) showed at least some improvement in the AAO-HNS functional disability rating, one-third of the labyrinthectomy group showed no improvement. The labyrinthectomy group was also more likely to rate their current imbalance as extremely or quite severe and to rate imbalance as interfering more often than the TLVNS group. The majority (>80%) of both subgroups had complete control of vertigo spells (Class A). These findings are in accordance with the literature showing that although the symptom of vertigo can be treated by a transmastoid labyrinthectomy, there is often persisting postoperative disequilibrium.[13,15]

When comparing Meniere's disease versus other diagnoses, the majority of both subgroups had good vertigo treatment class results (Class A or B), but current imbalance was rated as extremely severe or quite severe significantly less often in the

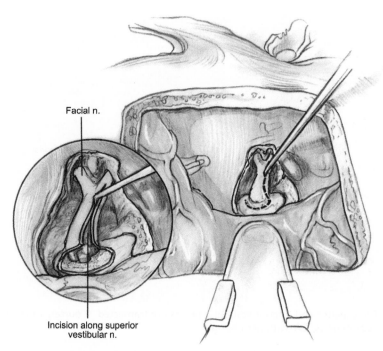

Facial n.

Incision along superior
vestibular n.

Fig. 17. The dura of the internal auditory canal is incised along the posterior aspect. (*From* Shelton C, Brackmann DE, House WF. Middle fossa approach. In: Brackmann DE, Shelton C, Arriaga MA, editors. Otologic surgery. 2nd edition. Philadelphia: WB Saunders; 2001. p. 503–10; with permission.)

Meniere's group, with ratings of the current frequency and severity of imbalance significantly better in the Meniere's group. Surgical procedures for vertigo appear to produce better results when there is a clear diagnosis of vertigo caused by Meniere's disease.

Based on subject ratings, surgery improved vertigo frequency, severity, interference, and AAO-HNS disability in all 3 surgical groups and improved imbalance for the ES and VNS groups. Vertigo spells are not the only source of discomfort to patients with peripheral vestibular disorders; imbalance also impacts quality of life and is likely to remain after surgery for vertigo.

Results of the first study suggested a possible difference in the postoperative outcome between labyrinthectomy and translabyrinthine vestibular nerve section (TLVNS), with labyrinthectomy having poorer results for imbalance (unsteadiness) though not for vertigo control. A second study was conducted to build on the findings of the authors' first study and to determine whether cutting the vestibular nerve (TLVNS) improves clinical outcomes beyond labyrinthectomy alone.[20] The same questionnaire used in the previous study was sent to subjects to assess symptom characteristics, including frequency, severity, interference, and amount of disability for both vertigo and disequilibrium before and after surgery, and the postoperative time course of improvements. Subject perceptions of the characteristics of their dizziness symptoms were compared between subjects undergoing labyrinthectomy and TLVNS.

The transmastoid labyrinthectomy allows for the complete removal of all neuroepithelial elements of the ear causing disabling disequilibrium, but at the expense of any remaining cochlear function. It was first described near the turn of the twentieth century and became accepted for relief of vertigo in the 1950s.[5–8]

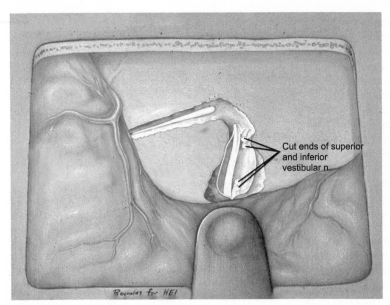

Cut ends of superior
and inferior
vestibular n.

Reynolds for HEI

Fig. 18. The superior and inferior vestibular nerves are transected. (*Courtesy of* House Ear Institute. Los Angeles, CA; with permission.)

William House popularized TLVNS in the late 1950s, and it has been called the gold standard for denervation procedures.[21] Nelson[21] notes that "It is both a postganglionic nerve section, because of the labyrinthectomy used to access the IAC, and a preganglionic procedure, because of the nerve section." TLVNS has been widely recommended as an excellent choice for the cure of disabling vertigo.[22,23]

The labyrinthectomy is a simpler procedure than the TLVNS and has been reported to have a good to excellent success rate for the cure of episodic vertigo.[15,17,24] However, there is incomplete removal of vestibular tissue with a labyrinthectomy because Scarpa's ganglion is not removed. It has been shown that this remaining tissue is capable of neuroma formation and may act as functional vestibular tissue capable of producing recurrent or persistent vertigo.[25–28] A TLVNS does remove Scarpa's ganglion and therefore assures the complete removal of all vestibular function. However, there are few reports in the literature to support the viewpoint that sectioning of the vestibular nerve is also necessary despite the adequate removal of all of the vestibular neuroepithelium.

Among 25 subjects who underwent transmastoid labyrinthectomies and 17 who underwent TLVNS, approximately 24% of each group still had vertigo (spinning dizziness). On average, both groups indicated resolution of vertigo at 2 to 3 weeks, and longer for imbalance. There were no significant differences between groups in vertigo characteristics, but TLVNS did show advantages in imbalance outcomes. AAO-HNS functional disability showed improvement in 73% and 52% of the TLVNS and labyrinthectomy groups, respectively. The TLVNS group was more likely to have improved imbalance (81.3% vs 45.8%, $P \leq .047$) and tended more frequently to rate it as currently not severe/none (76.5% vs 45.8%, $P \leq .06$). The labyrinthectomy group did not show significant improvement in any imbalance characteristics, whereas the TLVNS group improved in all characteristics. When limited to subjects with Meniere's disease, results are similar but differences between groups are smaller and improvement in imbalance did also occur for the labyrinthectomy group. These results led the authors to conclude that both transmastoid labyrinthectomy and TLVNS provide good control of vertigo (>85% Class A or B). However, subjects undergoing TLVNS were more likely to show improvement in imbalance and functional disability. This difference was less pronounced in subjects with Meniere's disease.

Because some subjects in every group (endolymphatic sac shunt, vestibular nerve section, and labyrinthectomy) in the first study reported still experiencing vertigo or spinning dizziness, and because subjects with labyrinthectomy and translabyrinthine VNS in the second study continued to experience severe vertigo and imbalance, a third study was conducted.[29] Possible reasons for failure of surgical procedures for vertigo have been suggested.[18,19] Surgical, diagnostic (peripheral vs central dizziness), and physiological (traumatic neuroma) mechanisms have been proposed. The study explored subject characteristics that might predict outcomes and help in preoperative or immediate postoperative counseling regarding expectations and control of vertigo or disequilibrium.

Primary outcomes included AAO-HNS vertigo score and class, number of spells per month, current and change in AAO-HNS disability rating, vertigo and imbalance severity ratings, and frequency of imbalance. The authors found that 3 preoperative factors were consistently related to outcome: AAO-HNS disability rating, imbalance frequency rating, and duration of first symptom (Rhos from 0.19–0.51, all $P < .05$). Greater disability and more frequent imbalance related to poorer outcome; but longer duration of disease related to better outcome. Presurgery vertigo characteristics were generally not related to outcome. Subjects with Meniere's disease were more likely to have improvement in imbalance as were those with no other significant disease and no allergy. Presence of tinnitus in the contralateral ear was associated with poorer outcomes, including a lower rate of Class A to B results ($P = .023$). Vertigo as a first symptom, contralateral tinnitus, and presence of eye disease also showed relationships to poorer outcome. The authors concluded that subjects rating themselves as more disabled before surgery are less likely to achieve the best outcomes, whereas frequency and severity of preoperative vertigo are not predictive.

SUMMARY

Several surgical approaches are performed to control the symptoms of peripheral vestibular disorders refractory to medical treatment. Surgery is usually reserved for patients with disabling vertigo. Surgery improves vertigo in endolymphatic sac shunts, vestibular nerve sections, and labyrinthectomies, and improves imbalance for the endolymphatic sac shunt and vestibular nerve section groups. Labyrinthectomy and TLVNS both offer excellent control of intractable vertigo. Persistent postoperative disequilibrium occurs at significant rates with both procedures, but is improved compared to preoperative ratings in the majority of patients who undergo a TLVNS. However, imbalance often does not improve and frequently worsens after a labyrinthectomy, which is more likely for diagnoses other than Meniere's disease. Finally, those rating themselves as more disabled before surgery are less likely to achieve the best outcomes.

REFERENCES

1. Jackler RK, Whinney D. A century of eighth nerve surgery. Otol Neurotol 2001;22: 401–16.
2. Silverstein H, Norrell H. Retrolabyrinthine surgery: a direct approach to the cerebellopontine angle. Otolaryngol Head Neck Surg 1980;88:462–9.

3. Silverstein H, Norrell H, Haberkamp T. A comparison of retrosigmoid IAC, retrolabyrinthine, and middle fossa vestibular neurectomy for treatment of vertigo. Laryngoscope 1987;97:165–73.
4. Silverstein H, Norrell H, Smouha EE. Retrosigmoid-internal auditory canal approach vs. retrolabyrinthine approach for vestibular neurectomy. Otolaryngol Head Neck Surg 1987;97:300–7.
5. Lake R. Removal of the semicircular canals in a case of unilateral aural vertigo. Lancet 1904;1:1567–8.
6. Cawthorne TE. The treatment of Ménière's disease. J Laryngol Otol 1943;58:363–71.
7. Day KM. Surgical treatment of hydrops of the labyrinth. Laryngoscope 1952;62:547–55.
8. Day KM. Labyrinth surgery for Ménière's disease. Laryngoscope 1943;53:617–30.
9. Portmann G. The saccus endolymphaticus and an operation for draining the same for the relief of vertigo. Arch Otolaryngol 1927;6:309.
10. House WF. Subarachnoid shunt for drainage of endolymphatic hydrops. Laryngoscope 1962;72:713–29.
11. Telischi FF, Luxford WM. Long-term efficacy of endolymphatic sac surgery for vertigo in Menière's disease. Otolaryngol Head Neck Surg 1993;109:83–7.
12. Shelton C, Brackmann DE, House WF. Middle fossa approach. In: Brackmann DE, Shelton C, Arriaga MA, editors. Otologic surgery. 2nd edition. Philadelphia: WB Saunders; 2001. p. 503–10.
13. Garcia-Ibanez E, Garcia-Ibanez JL. Middle fossa vestibular neurectomy: a report of 373 cases. Otolaryngol Head Neck Surg 1980;88:486–90.
14. De la Cruz A, Teufert KB, Berliner KI. Surgical treatment for vertigo: patient survey of vertigo, imbalance, and time course for recovery. Otolaryngol Head Neck Surg 2006;135:541–8.
15. Glasscock ME 3rd, Hughes GB, Davis WE, et al. Labyrinthectomy versus middle fossa vestibular nerve section in Meniere's disease. A critical evaluation of relief of vertigo. Ann Otol Rhinol Laryngol 1980;89:318–24.
16. Schuknecht HF. Behavior of the vestibular nerve following labyrinthectomy. Ann Otol Rhinol Laryngol Suppl 1982;97:16–32.
17. Kemink JL, Telian SA, Graham MD, et al. Transmastoid labyrinthectomy: reliable surgical management of vertigo. Otolaryngol Head Neck Surg 1989;101:5–10.
18. Thedinger BS, Thedinger BA. Analysis of patients with persistent dizziness after vestibular nerve section. Ear Nose Throat J 1998;77:290–2.
19. Moon IS, Hain TC. Delayed quick spins after vestibular nerve section respond to anticonvulsant therapy. Otol Neurotol 2005;26:82–5.
20. De la Cruz A, Teufert KB, Berliner KI. Transmastoid labyrinthectomy versus translabyrinthine vestibular nerve section: does cutting the nerve make a difference in outcome? Otol Neurotol 2007;28:801–8.
21. Nelson RA. Translabyrinthine vestibular neurectomy. In: Brackmann DE, Shelton C, Arriaga MA, editors. Otologic surgery. 2nd edition. Philadelphia: WB Saunders; 2001. p. 433–9.
22. Brackmann DE. Vestibular nerve section: translabyrinthine approach. Oper Tech Otolaryngol Head Neck Surg 1991;2:28–31.
23. Nelson RA. Surgery for control of vertigo. In: Wiet RJ, Cause JB, editors, Complications in otolaryngology - head and neck surgery. Ear and skull base, vol. 1. Philadelphia: BC Decker; 1986. p. 149–59.

24. Pulec JL. Labyrinthectomy: indications, technique and results. Laryngoscope 1974;84:1552–73.
25. Linthicum FH Jr, Alonso A, Denia A. Traumatic neuroma: a complication of transcanal labyrinthectomy. Arch Otolaryngol 1979;105:654–5.
26. Ylikoski J, Belal A Jr. Human vestibular nerve morphology and labyrinthectomy. Am J Otolaryngol 1981;2:81–93.
27. Jung TT, Anderson JH, Paparella MM. Cochleovestibular nerve sections in labyrinthectomized patients. Am J Otol 1987;8:155–8.
28. Monsell EM, Brackmann DE, Linthicum FH Jr. Why do vestibular destructive procedures sometimes fail? Otolaryngol Head Neck Surg 1988;99:472–9.
29. Teufert KB, Berliner KI, De la Cruz A. Persistent dizziness after surgical treatment of vertigo: an exploratory study of prognostic factors. Otol Neurotol 2007;28: 1056–62.

Early Vestibular Physical Therapy Rehabilitation for Meniere's Disease

Kim R. Gottshall, PhD[a], Shelby G. Topp, MD[b],
Michael E. Hoffer, MD[a],*

KEYWORDS

• Meniere's disease • Vestibular rehabilitation
• Vestibular therapy • Vestibular physical therapy

The treatment of Meniere's disease remains one of the most controversial areas in the field of otolaryngology. Although there have been significant advances in surgical and minimally invasive therapy over the years, there is still no consensus on therapeutic options, especially after conservative medical therapy fails. In an attempt to provide the best and most conservative care there has been a great deal of interest in the use of vestibular physical therapy rehabilitation in Meniere's treatment. To examine this topic in more detail, we consider some basic information about vestibular physical therapy rehabilitation and then examine the role of vestibular physical therapy rehabilitation in Meniere's disease as it currently is used. Last, we examine the prospect of initiating rehabilitation earlier in the time course of the disease.

VESTIBULAR PHYSICAL THERAPY REHABILITATION

The goal of a vestibular physical therapy rehabilitation program (VR) is to decrease dizziness, improve gaze stabilization, improve postural stability, and enhance general

---

Disclosure Statements: I am a military service member. This work was prepared as part of my official duties. Title 17 U.S.C. 105 provides that "Copyright protection under this title is not available for any work of the United States Government." Title 17 U.S.C. 101 defines a United States Government work as a work prepared by a military service member or employee of the United States Government as part of that person's official duties.
"The views expressed in this article are those of the author(s) and do not necessarily reflect the official policy or position of the Department of the Navy, Department of Defense, or the United States Government."
[a] Department of Otolaryngology, Naval Medical Center San Diego, Spatial Orientation Center, 34520 Bob Wilson Drive, Suite 200, San Diego, CA 92134, USA
[b] Department of Otolaryngology, Naval Medical Center San Diego, 34520 Bob Wilson Drive, Suite 200, San Diego, CA 92134, USA
* Corresponding author.
E-mail address: Michael.hoffer@med.navy.mil

Otolaryngol Clin N Am 43 (2010) 1113–1119
doi:10.1016/j.otc.2010.05.006
0030-6665/10/$ – see front matter. Published by Elsevier Inc.

function in the activities of daily living and work. Physical therapists conduct vestibular function tests and based on the differential diagnosis choose specific exercises designed to decrease dizziness, increase balance function, and increase general activity levels customized to the individual patient. Vestibular compensation occurs as the plasticity of the central nervous system is specifically activated and established or redundant pathways are accessed. Vestibular physical therapy engages active head movement in concert with processing of visual, vestibular, and somatosensory stimuli to drive a progressive decrease in symptoms of dizziness or disequilibrium. Peripheral vestibular compensation may involve recovery of vestibulo-ocular reflex (VOR) gain or adaptation exercises. Habituation may require exercises to decrease dizziness by focusing on exposure to a specific stimulus for attenuation of the dizziness response in the brain. Substitution strategies may be implemented in those patients with complete loss of peripheral vestibular function. Balance retraining may require an array of exercises designed to improve organization of sensory information for postural control and coordination of muscle responses. General activity exercise to elevate functional endurance may involve a daily aerobic exercise program of progressive walking, cycling, or swimming.

THE ROLE OF VESTIBULAR PHYSICAL THERAPY REHABILITATION IN MENIERE'S DISEASE
Vestibular Rehabilitation After Destructive Procedures

Meniere's disease is a common disorder that has a classical presentation including fluctuating hearing loss, tinnitus, and ear pressure with episodic vertigo episodes. Although a great deal of work has focused on these symptoms, little attention has been directed at other functional disabilities associated with Meniere's disease. In particular, individuals with chronic Meniere's disease often develop symptoms of unsteadiness and disability.[1] These are symptoms that have been shown to respond to vestibular physical therapy intervention in other vestibulopathies.[2] However, little work has been done documenting the use of physical therapy in Meniere's disease except for its use after definitive destructive therapy.[3–5] One area where rehabilitation has an established role in the therapy for Meniere's disease is after vestibular neurectomy or labyrinthectomy. In both cases, the surgical procedure creates a fixed and complete unilateral vestibular loss. This sudden vestibular deafferentation may produce a significant amount of unsteadiness. The amount of unsteadiness will be dependent on the amount of vestibular function that was present before the surgical procedure. Those who had the most function will generally have the greatest degree of dysfunction after ablation surgery. Prior evidence to support the advantages of rehabilitation after destructive surgery comes mostly from the acoustic neuroma literature. A number of groups have shown improved outcomes in terms of time to recovery using vestibular physical therapy rehabilitation instituted early after translabyrinthine tumor resection.[2,6–8] Although the disorders are not the same, the end result of complete loss of unilateral vestibular function allows for the conclusion that, like patients undergoing translabyrinthine excision of acoustic neuromas, those undergoing vestibular deafferentation via labyrinthectomy or nerve section with Meniere's disease should also benefit from early therapy. It can then be surmised that after destructive procedures for Meniere's disease, vestibular rehabilitation therapy should demonstrate efficacy in the speed of recovery and postural stability. Therefore, in many centers, vestibular physical therapy rehabilitation after destructive procedures is the accepted best practice for ensuring decreased postural sway and improved daily function for patients with Meniere's disease. Results indicate that customized vestibular, visual, and somatosensory training hasten adaptive processes. Sensory conflicts are resolved more efficiently, resulting in a reduction of disequilibrium within 3 weeks. There is evidence this postural stability prevails months later.[9]

Vestibular Rehabilitation After Vertigo Resolution

Another logical use of vestibular physical therapy rehabilitation is in individuals in which episodic vertigo has abated without a surgical or chemical ablative intervention, but disequilibrium persists. Clendaniel and Tucci[1] demonstrated the value of a defined exercise program in treating this "postvertigo" disequilibrium. Much like using vestibular physical therapy rehabilitation in the postoperative patient, using rehabilitation to treat chronic unsteadiness is consistent with other proven instances in which vestibular physical therapy rehabilitation has been successful.

Work in our lab confirms Clendaniel and Tucci's findings.[10] Patients presenting to our tertiary care center with symptoms of Meniere's disease were eligible to enroll in a study approved by the Institutional Review Board. Subjects underwent a history and standardized physical examination, as well as a complete auditory-vestibular test battery that included rotational chair testing (Micromedical, Chatham, IL, USA) and computerized dynamic posturography (CDP) (Neurocom Inc, Clackamas, OR, USA).[11] The patients also underwent a set of vestibular functional tasks to measure balance function. These tests included Romberg, tandem Romberg, tandem gait, gait with head motion, head thrusts, headshake dynamic visual acuity, Fukuda step tests, and 3 standard cerebellar tests. Patients who demonstrated abnormal function in any of the vestibular testing procedures, complained of disequilibrium or unsteadiness, and had episodic vertigo were treated with medication to control vertigo. When patients reported no vertigo attacks for at least 3 months they were further assessed and entered in a vestibular physical therapy rehabilitation program. The Dizziness Handicap Index (DHI),[12] Activities Balance Confidence Scale (ABC),[13] Dynamic Gait Index (DGI),[14] and computerized dynamic posturography (CDP) sensory organization test (SOT) were administered as vestibular physical therapy intake and outcome measures.

Vestibular physical therapy exercises targeted VOR, cervico-ocular reflex (COR), depth perception (DP), somatosensory retraining (SS), and aerobic function. The VOR, COR, and DP exercises were graded in difficulty based on velocity of head and object motion and by progression of body positioning from sitting to standing to walking. The SS exercises were graded in difficulty by narrowing the base of support, making the surface uneven, or changing the surface from firm to soft. Varied walking exercises were graded in difficulty by changing direction, requiring performance with the eyes closed, increasing speed of ambulation, walking on soft surfaces, or navigating stairs. An aerobic exercise home program progressively increased the time, speed, or distance that the patient could tolerate. Patients were treated once a week for 8 weeks. In 1 year, 26 individuals met criteria for inclusion in the study. All outcome measures showed significant improvement with significance defined as P less than .05. CDP SOT score improved from 51.1 before therapy to 68.5 after therapy. The results for the remaining 3 outcome measures also approached significance and are shown in **Fig. 1**. The DGI nearly normalized with a group mean of 23.2 of a possible 24 at the end of therapy.

This Meniere's study showed the benefit of postvertigo resolution vestibular physical therapy rehabilitation. Our population was composed exclusively of those with unilateral Meniere's; therefore, we can make no conclusion regarding bilateral disease. In fact, Cohen[15] noted that in bilateral disease vestibular physical therapy rehabilitation is not effective and advocated adaptive strategies (eg, equipment) for this patient population.

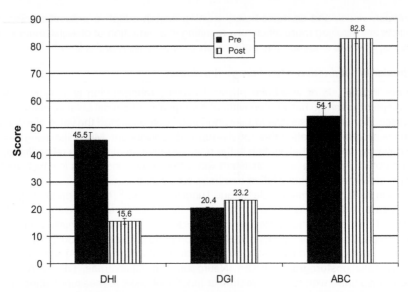

Fig. 1. Outcome after 8 weeks of vestibular rehabilitation in patients who had no vertigo attacks for at least 3 months before starting therapy.

NEW FRONTIERS

To date, the established role of vestibular physical therapy rehabilitation in Meniere's disease is to treat disequilibrium secondary to surgical ablation or after vertigo episodes subside. There are 2 other instances in the treatment of Meniere's disease in which treatment might be considered: (1) after treatment has stopped or significantly reduced the vertigo where constant disequilibrium is disabling and (2) in patients with active fluctuating disease. Our group has published data examining the effects of vestibular physical therapy rehabilitation therapy in individuals undergoing transtympanic gentamicin therapy. Although there are many reports that transtympanic treatment is associated with a high rate of posttreatment disequilibrium, our data examine long-term results in a group of treated patients with little posttreatment (postgentamicin) unsteadiness.[16] In our long-term data we examined a group of 25 individuals all of whom underwent microcatheter-administered gentamicin to treat intractable dizziness 8 to 10 years before the follow-up assessment. In that study cohort, 14 patients had not undergone rehabilitation and 11 had undergone rehabilitation immediately after microcatheter treatment. We had previously shown that at 2 years the rehabilitation group had significantly better CDP SOT scores than the nonrehabilitation group. All 25 individuals were available for follow-up. Once again, group mean scores on CDP SOT, DGI, DHI, and ABC were used for comparison. Even 8 to 10 years after therapy, the rehabilitation group fared better than the nonrehabilitation group. The CDP SOT difference was significant at P less than .05, whereas the remaining data approached significance in all cases. The results for the remaining outcome measures are shown in **Fig. 2**. These data, then, argue that rehabilitation has a role as an adjuvant to ablative Meniere's treatment and this value persists long term.

We have recently begun to look at a group of patients undergoing rehabilitation before the resolution of vertigo episodes and before the initiation of any therapy beyond diet and medication. Many individuals with Meniere's disease experience some degree of unsteadiness between attacks. We predict that these individuals

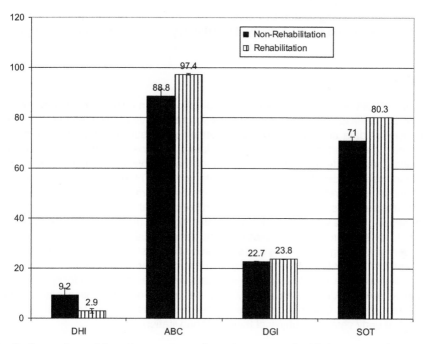

Fig. 2. Comparison of long-term outcome in patients treated with intratympanic genta-micin therapy who underwent 8 weeks of vestibular rehabilitation versus a group that did not undergo rehabilitation.

will benefit from therapy. Vestibular physical therapy rehabilitation may have several goals in this group of patients. Beyond treating the unsteadiness, exercises may be designed to decrease anxiety and improve confidence in performing functional daily or work tasks. The achievement of short-term vestibular goals provides the therapist treating the patient with useful measures to assess patient progress and design the next tier of treatment. Nevertheless, it is possible that with the balance function of one ear fluctuating over time, vestibular physical therapy rehabilitation will not change unsteadiness experienced during vertigo attacks.

Currently, we are examining the impact of early vestibular physical therapy rehabil-itation on the vertigo episodes in a group of patients with Meniere's disease. Tradi-tional teaching is that vestibular physical therapy rehabilitation is ineffective in those patients with episodic vertigo. However, our lab and other groups have demonstrated the utility of vestibular physical therapy rehabilitation for the largely fluctuating symp-toms seen in migraine-associated dizziness (MAD).[17] The pathology and symptom-atology of MAD is distinct from that of endolymphatic hydrops. Patients with migraines undergo less fluctuation of balance function, but do show subtle abnormal-ities even between attacks on objective testing. In contrast, patients with Meniere's disease have significant changes in balance function during vertigo attacks to include crisis of Tumarkin and often experience subtle unsteadiness between symptoms. However, there is likely a subset of patients with Meniere's disease who will respond to vestibular physical therapy rehabilitation with measurable resiliency to the onset of episodic vertigo. Optimizing spatial orientation strategies and decreasing anxiety might be viable options as additional patient tools in the treatment of Meniere's disease. Documenting vestibular characteristics by testing of responders and nonresponders before and after several weeks of therapy is an ongoing focus of study in our clinic.

SUMMARY

The use of vestibular physical therapy rehabilitation as an adjuvant in the treatment of Meniere's disease has now been in place for several years. Nevertheless, there is a paucity of data and published work examining this subject. It is clear both from Meniere's data, and from unilateral and bilateral peripheral vestibular hypofunction physical therapy literature, that rehabilitation has a role in treating dizziness and unsteadiness that develops after ablative intervention. There are also data to support the routine use of rehabilitation after transtympanic therapy in individuals who show subtle unsteadiness. The use of rehabilitation in individuals with Meniere's disease still experiencing active vertigo attacks is a fascinating area that still requires further clarification. By extension from success of vestibular physical therapy in treating patients with vertiginous migraines there is a suggestion that vestibular physical therapy may be beneficial in treating Meniere's unsteadiness between vertigo attacks. Increasing the resilience of the somatosensory, visual, and vestibular integration for spatial orientation as well as decreasing anxiety may be useful tools for these patients with Meniere's disease. Continued studies are needed in this realm to truly delineate the benefit of early vestibular physical therapy rehabilitation.

REFERENCES

1. Clendaniel RA, Tucci DL. Vestibular rehabilitation strategies in Meniere's disease. Otolaryngol Clin North Am 1997;30(6):1145–58.
2. Herdman SJ. Role of vestibular adaptation in vestibular physical therapy rehabilitation. Otolaryngol Head Neck Surg 1998;119(1):49–54.
3. Odkvist L. Gentamicin cures vertigo, but what happens to hearing. Int Tinnitus J 1997;3(2):133–6.
4. Gottshall KR, Hoffer ME, Kopke RD, et al. Vestibular physical therapy rehabilitation after low dose microcatheter administered gentamicin treatment for Meniere's disease. In: Proceedings of the 4th International Symposium on Meniere's disease. Hague (The Netherlands): Kuglar Publications; 2000. p. 663–8.
5. Suryanarayanan R, Cook JA. Long-term results of gentamicin inner ear perfusion in Meniere's disease. J Laryngol Otol 2004;118(7):489–95.
6. Vereeck L, Wuyts FL, Truijen S, et al. The effect of early customized vestibular physical therapy rehabilitation on balance after acoustic neuroma resection. Clin Rehabil 2008;22(8):698–713.
7. Enticott JC, O'leary SJ, Briggs RJ. Effects of vestibulo-ocular reflex exercises on vestibular compensation after vestibular schwannoma surgery. Otol Neurotol 2005;26(2):265–9.
8. Tjernström F, Fransson PA, Kahlon B, et al. Vestibular PREHAB and gentamicin before schwannoma surgery may improve long-term postural function. J Neurol Neurosurg Psychiatr 2009;80(11):1254–60.
9. Magnusson M, Kahlon B, Karlberg M, et al. Vestibular "PREHAB". Ann N Y Acad Sci 2009;1164:257–62.
10. Gottshall KR, Hoffer ME, Moore RJ, et al. The role of vestibular physical therapy rehabilitation in the treatment of Meniere's disease. Otolaryngol Head Neck Surg 2005;133(3):326–8.

11. Norre ME. Relevance of function tests in the diagnosis of vestibular disorders. Clin Otolaryngol 1994;19(5):433–40.
12. Jacobson GP, Newman CW. The development of the dizziness handicap inventory. Arch Otolaryngol Head Neck Surg 1990;116:424–7.
13. Powell LE, Meyers AM. The activities-specific balance confidence scale. J Gerontol Med Sci 1995;50(1):28–34.
14. Shumway-Cook A, Woolacott M. Motor control theory and practical applications. Baltimore (MD): Williams and Wilkins; 1995.
15. Cohen H. Vestibular physical therapy rehabilitation improves daily life function. Am J Occup Ther 1994;48(10):919–25.
16. Gottshall KR, Hoffer ME, Moore RJ. Long-term impact of vestibular physical therapy rehabilitation after gentamicin therapy in the outcome of Meniere's disease. In: Presented at the 30th mid winter meeting of the Association for Research in Otolaryngology. Denver (CO), February 10–15, 2007.
17. Gottshall KR, Moore RH, Hoffer ME. Vestibular physical therapy rehabilitation for migraine-associated dizziness. Int Tinnitus J 2005;11(1):81–4.

Genetic Investigations of Meniere's Disease

Jeffrey T. Vrabec, MD

KEYWORDS

• Meniere's disease • Gene • Etiology • Pathogenesis

DEFINITION

Meniere's disease (MD) is a clinical disorder defined by the symptom complex of fluctuating sensorineural hearing loss, vertigo, tinnitus, and aural pressure. In an effort to develop uniform reporting criteria for MD, the American Academy of Otolaryngology-Head and Neck Surgery (AAO-HNS) Committee on Hearing and Equilibrium published guidelines for diagnosing this entity in 1995.[1] To be diagnosed with definite MD, a patient must display two or more episodes of characteristic vertigo (each episode lasting longer than 20 minutes), documented hearing loss (typically fluctuating low-frequency sensorineural loss seen on serial audiograms), and presence of aural pressure or tinnitus in the affected ear, and other causes of vertigo must be excluded. The effort to include only definite cases in clinical studies of MD is intended to allow reliable comparisons among different institutions. Not all patients presenting to specialty clinics will satisfy diagnostic criteria for definite MD, because isolated hearing symptoms are common. In general, approximately two-thirds of patients with symptoms of MD will be classified as definite, whereas the remainder are usually classified as possible MD.[2,3]

The natural history of MD has been documented in several studies.[4–6] The mean age of onset is between 45 and 55 years. Sensorineural hearing loss typically begins in low frequencies, and will show fluctuation early in the disease. With time, fluctuation ceases and most patients develop a progressive moderate to severe hearing loss. The hearing tends to stabilize 8 to 10 years after onset.[7] Vertigo symptoms are dramatic at onset, but also tend to diminish in frequency and severity over time. Vestibular function usually remains compromised in the affected ear. The disorder is unilateral at onset in most cases, but with extended follow-up, symptoms may develop in the opposite ear in up to 30% of patients. The list of treatment options is extensive. The general tendency toward diminished vertigo attacks, reports of similar efficacy for

Bobby R. Alford Department of Otolaryngology – Head and Neck Surgery Baylor College of Medicine, 6550 Fannin Street, SM1727, Houston, TX 77030, USA
E-mail address: jvrabec@bcm.edu

Otolaryngol Clin N Am 43 (2010) 1121–1132
doi:10.1016/j.otc.2010.05.010
0030-6665/10/$ – see front matter © 2010 Elsevier Inc. All rights reserved.

oto.theclinics.com

widely varying treatment modalities, paucity of controlled studies, and inability to alter the progression of hearing loss casts doubt on the ultimate value of medical management.[8-10] Clearly, greater understanding of the pathophysiology of this disorder would enhance clinical management.

ETIOLOGY/PATHOGENESIS

Endolymphatic hydrops has been consistently identified as a histologic feature of temporal bone specimens from patients with MD. Historically, great significance was attached to this finding, resulting in speculation that hydrops produced the characteristic symptoms of MD. More recent analysis of temporal bone specimens by Merchant and colleagues[11] described similar degrees of endolymphatic hydrops in specimens from people with and without the characteristic symptoms of MD. However, patients with MD who did not have hydrops on histologic examination have also been reported, and therefore the presence of hydrops is neither essential nor specific to MD. The event that triggers development of hydrops remains undefined, although disruption of Na+/K+ homeostasis may be an important contributing factor.[12]

Numerous theories regarding MD pathogenesis exist, with it being broadly categorized as caused by metabolic, autonomic, or endocrine dysfunction; allergy; autoimmunity; trauma; infectious disease; or vascular disease. Each theory has varying degrees of supportive evidence. Some preliminary observations have not been replicated in subsequent studies, illustrated by the ambiguity of the role of autoimmunity in MD.[13,14] The relative contributions of each potential theory may be predicted based partially on clinical history. Trauma and acute infectious events are rarely associated with the development of symptoms. The typically unilateral symptoms are difficult to explain based on a theory of systemic metabolic, endocrine, allergic, immune, or vascular disorders. Finally, little epidemiologic evidence shows that other comorbid diseases exceed the expected population prevalence in patients with MD, with the possible exception of migraine.[15] Although none of the proposed theories can be categorically rejected, two interesting possibilities that do account for the unilateral nature of the disease are migraine and recrudescent viral infection.

Vestibular symptoms are frequently described in individuals with migraine. The diagnostic criteria for migraine-associated dizziness are fulfillment of International Headache Society (IHS) criteria for migraine headache with concurrent vestibular symptoms.[16] These individuals rarely have any associated hearing loss.[17] Other experts have observed that the prevalence of migraine in patients with MD exceeds that of the expected population prevalence. The highest percentage of concomitant MD and migraine is reported to be 56% of all patients with MD.[18] This finding suggests that MD attacks and migraine headache share a common pathway for symptom development. Additional support is provided by the clinical observation that agents for migraine prophylaxis have shown benefit in some patients with MD.[19]

The genetic component of migraine is clinically evident and partially defined at the molecular level. At least nine loci exist for common migraine with or without aura, and three for familial hemiplegic migraine (FHM). Mutations in three different genes are described for different pedigrees of FHM.[20] All of these, *CACNA1A, ATP1A2,* and *SCN1A*, code for intracellular ion channels. Rapid changes in intracellular electrolyte concentrations are suspected to take place in the presence of a dysfunctional ion channel. This mechanism remains appealing as a potential explanation for the episodic vertigo and fluctuating hearing loss characteristic of MD.

The possibility of a viral infection is considered because of the ubiquitous presence and ease of transmission of the potential infectious agents. However, the inaccessibility of the labyrinth for routine culture and variable systemic immune response make clinical confirmation of a viral infection difficult. The recurrent nature of symptoms in patients with MD favors a virus that is capable of recrudescence, rather than repeated inoculation of virus from an external source.[21]

Herpes viruses, including herpes simplex virus (HSV) and varicella zoster virus (VZV), are neurotrophic DNA viruses capable of establishing a latent infection in sensory nerve ganglia. Reactivation of the virus and resulting viral replication induces an inflammatory response with clinical symptoms depending on the specific nerve involved. Intermittent symptoms interspersed within periods of quiescence, recurrence provoked by stress, variable severity, and a tendency for symptoms to decrease with extended follow-up are all characteristic of both MD and HSV reactivation.[6,22,23]

GENETIC BASIS FOR MENIERE'S DISEASE

An attractive method for corroborating any given theory of MD pathogenesis (autoimmune disease, migraine variant, herpes virus infection) is through genetic investigation. Defining a gene mutation that determines susceptibility would obviously support a given theory and refocus treatment efforts on a specific molecular pathway. The search for a genetic contribution to any disease process involves careful epidemiologic study of the target population. Clinical observations regarding the prevalence, age of onset, gender, race, socioeconomic status, familial tendency, and comorbid conditions help in formulating a hypothesis of disease susceptibility. Objective data that can be used to confirm the diagnosis enhance the ability to define affected individuals.

Several features of MD suggest a genetic component. A distinct racial predilection is recognized. The prevalence is highest in Caucasians, with an estimated 218 cases per 100,000 persons.[5,24] Familial cases of MD were first reported by Brown in 1941, with an estimated 7% of all patients having affected family members.[24,25] Siblings of patients display a 10-fold increased risk of developing the disease.[26] Several MD pedigrees have been reported, mostly in Caucasians.[24,27–31] Several Brazilian families with concurrent MD and migraine are also described.[32] The larger series of patients indicate that familial MD is inherited in an autosomal dominant manner with an estimated penetrance of 60%.[24,31,33]

LINKAGE STUDIES

Classical genetic investigation focused on collecting a group of people with a similar genetic background, some of whom expressed a trait or disease of interest and some that did not. Analysis of an extended family pedigree allows geneticists to analyze methods of inheritance and penetrance of a given genetic disorder. With this information in hand, the genomes of the affected individuals are compared with the controls to assess for regions that are distinctly different in the disease group.

Analysis with sets of genomic markers that are progressively closer together improves the resolution of the region of interest, leading to identification of a candidate gene. Sequencing of the candidate gene ultimately identifies mutations that alter gene function, confirming the gene's role in disease development. The method is particularly robust for single genes with large effect, in which mutation of a single gene product or function results in a readily discernable alteration in anatomy or function of a single or multiple organ systems. Pedigree studies have identified most of the currently recognized syndromes of hereditary hearing loss.[34] In several of these examples, insight into disease mechanisms was gained after identification of the responsible gene.

Genetic markers of MD have not been identified precisely. Several reported linkage sites as shown in **Table 1**. Early studies focused on analyzing human leukocyte antigens (HLAs), presuming dysfunction in immune function or autoimmunity as a factor in disease development. Among the earliest studies, an association was detected between the Cw7 antigen and MD.[35] Multiple studies have been performed since, with different HLA associations or no association reported by the various authors.[24,30,31,36,37] Both susceptibility and resistance antigens are purported. Only one study provides replication of the Cw7 association, with others contradicting this association.[38] The finding of a significant association in the HLA complex led to increased scrutiny of chromosome 6p as a candidate gene, although none has been identified.

Fransen and colleagues[39] recognized the presence of concurrent auditory and vestibular symptoms in a large Belgian family with hereditary hearing loss, designated DFNA9. The gene responsible for the disorder is cochlin (*COCH*). The presence of variable auditory and vestibular symptoms prompted the authors to suggest a relationship with MD. However, the clinical course of DFNA9 and MD are different. Some temporal bones from individuals with DFNA9 hearing loss have shown the presence of endolymphatic hydrops, but the characteristic finding in DFNA9 is microfibrillar deposits in the stria vascularis, a feature not detected in MD.[40] Individuals with DFNA9 develop hearing loss at a young age, the hearing loss is more often high frequency, the vestibular symptoms include chronic disequilibrium and oscillopsia, and both auditory and vestibular deficits progress to severe loss of function with advancing age. Subsequent studies of sporadic MD cases have failed to confirm any association of *COCH* with MD.[41] In addition, other familial cases of MD have not been associated with *COCH* mutations.[24,42]

Morrison and Johnson[24] propose a unique familial MD locus on chromosome 14q that is distinct from *COCH*. In their series, linkage data suggested a locus in a region overlapping *COCH*. However, mutation analysis did not detect any of the reported *COCH* mutations in DFNA9, or any novel mutations. They concluded that their familial locus is not in *COCH* but do not propose an alternative candidate gene.

A large Swedish family was studied for linkage to loci in known familial forms of cochleovestibular dysfunction, and using a genome wide set of microsatellite markers.[42,43] The investigators did not find any association with hereditary hearing loss loci for DFNA1, DFNA6/14, DFNA9, or DFNA15. This family did show linkage for several markers on chromosome 12. When combined with additional families, the locus was narrowed to 12p12.3. Within this region only a single known gene is identified, phosphoinositide-3-kinase (*PIK3C2G*). Mutation analysis involving the coding regions of the gene did not detect any mutations.

Lynch and colleagues[44] selected a candidate gene for mutation analysis from a series of familial MD cases. No preliminary linkage study was performed in this group

Table 1
Proposed Meniere's Disease loci

Location	Ethnic	Can Gene	Replication	Phenotype
12p12.3	Swedish	*PIK3C2G*	No	MD
14q11–13	UK	None	No	MD
COCH	Danish	*COCH*	No	Not MD
6p	Multiple	Hla region	No	MD

Abbreviations: Can Gene, candidate gene; MD, Meniere's disease.

of individuals; rather, the antiquin (*ATQ*) gene was selected based on a presumed effect in maintenance of fluid balance. Mhatre and colleagues[45] reported a similar "mutation analysis first" approach in unrelated patients with the aquaporin-2 (*AQP2*) gene. Proceeding straight to mutation analysis is inherently precarious, because it presupposes that the correct physiologic disruption producing the disease is known. Not surprisingly, no gene alterations unique to the patient group were identified in either study.

ANIMAL MODELS

No evidence shows that MD will occur spontaneously in animals. The hallmark symptoms of the disease—recurrent vertigo and fluctuating sensorineural hearing loss in animals—are also difficult to produce in animals. Therefore, animal models have been designed to replicate the histologic feature of endolymphatic hydrops. This feature is most reliably produced by occluding the endolymphatic duct in the guinea pig, but the effects of the procedure are not uniform across species.[46] Multiple methods for inducing hydrops in animals are reported, although not as uniformly successful as the guinea pig model.

Although valuable for understanding changes in physiology caused by endolymphatic hydrops, therapeutic interventions are difficult to develop based on this model. Symptoms associated with the guinea pig hydrops model include some early fluctuating hearing loss, but minimal to no vestibular dysfunction is appreciated.[46,47]

Several rodent models develop endolymphatic hydrops as a consequence of single gene mutations such as *Slc26A4*, *Foxi1*, *Brn-4*, and *Phex*.[48–50] All are related to hereditary human hearing loss; Pendred syndrome and DFNB4 for *Slc26A4* and *Foxi1*, DFN3 for *Brn-4*(*POU3F4*), and familial hypophosphatemic rickets for *Phex*. Onset of hydrops is very early in all except *Phex*, where a progressive hearing loss and hydrops is seen. The clinical features in humans parallel the findings in the animal models; however, all are distinctly different from the presentation of MD (**Table 2**).

Congenital onset, radiographic evident of labyrinthine malformation, and mixed hearing loss distinguish the clinical presentation of Pendred syndrome, nonsyndromic enlarged vestibular aqueduct, and X-linked mixed deafness with stapes gusher. Vestibular symptoms may be present in any of these, although vertigo characteristic of MD is not likely. Several reports exist of hearing loss in familial hypophosphatemic rickets. Meisner and colleagues[51] summarized the reported hearing changes, indicating that hearing loss is rare in young patients, and predominantly high frequency. Vestibular symptoms are reported by some patients, but the available reports do not contain enough detail to determine if the vertigo is characteristic of MD or not.

Variable audiometric and vestibular findings in these animal models despite the histologic finding of endolymphatic hydrops illustrate the lack of specificity of hydrops

Table 2 Animal models manifesting endolymphatic hydrops				
Gene	**Hearing**	**Vestibular**	**Onset**	**Humans**
Phex	MHL	Yes	Adult	Rickets
Brn-4/POU3F4	MHL	No	Birth −/−, Adult ±	DFN3
Slc26a4	SNHL	No	Birth	DFNB4, Pendred
Foxi1	SNHL	No	Birth	

Abbreviations: MHL, mixed hearing loss; SNHL, sensorineural hearing loss; −/−, homozygous for the mutant allele; ±, heterozygous.

as a marker of the clinical symptoms of fluctuating hearing loss and episodic vertigo. The applicability of the animal models to MD is questionable because the human conditions represented are not clinically similar to MD. Thus, mutations of these genes are unlikely to contribute to development of sporadic MD. Ultimately, physiologic dysfunction that produces hydrops may have a similar common pathway of development; however, this mechanism remains obscure.

ASSOCIATION STUDIES FOR COMPLEX DISEASES

Linkage analysis is less successful for identifying complex diseases, those caused by gene interactions, or the combined effect of an environmental factor on a susceptible genetic background, because the gene or genes of interest may not be independently sufficient to produce the disease. It is increasingly likely that the genetic contribution in MD is complex. Association studies offer an alternative to linkage analysis.[52] Collections of individuals manifesting a common phenotype represent the study group. In practice, subject accrual for an association study is technically easier as it does not require the identification of a large pedigree with a high prevalence of the disease of interest. For genes with only a modest increased risk of disease, family based studies are impractical. Transmission disequilibrium testing using affected individuals and their parents is often recommended. However, even this approach becomes problematic when the disorder of interest is adult onset. Carefully selected case-control association studies allow a method for studying adult-onset complex diseases.[53]

Proliferation of both family-based and case-control association studies in recent years is largely caused by improved tools for genetic analysis. Definition of more than 3 million single nucleotide polymorphisms (SNPs) throughout the human genome provides markers for detailed analysis in any chromosomal region, predicting that an SNP likely exists in proximity (and high linkage disequilibrium) to the ultimate gene or mutation of interest. Measurement of linkage disequilibrium in Caucasian populations finds regions of high linkage disequilibrium averaging 10 kb in length adjacent to common alleles.[54] The combination of efficient techniques for high throughput genotyping with dense SNP maps offers a high level of definition for genome-wide studies. Constraints to genome-wide association are costs and evolving methods of statistical analysis.

Limitations of association studies in defining new disease genes are well recognized.[55] Inaccurate phenotype definition and overinterpretation of SNPs of only mildly increased risk can lead to premature claims of association. Replication of the association in a second population is essential to confirm any preliminary finding.[55] Some important methods to limit false-positive associations include matching cases and controls and pursuing genes of likely functional importance based on theories of disease pathogenesis.[56] Matching controls for ethnicity is essential given the variable marker allele frequencies in different populations, whereas matching for age, gender, or domicile may be recommended based on the clinical impressions of these variables on disease development. Matching controls that have also been excluded for the disease of interest using an objective measurement represent the ideal control group. Ultimately, the effect size of a given marker profoundly impacts the ease of identification, because the markers that confer a substantial risk increase can be identified with relatively small samples, whereas those with only modest risk will require very large sample sizes.[57]

CANDIDATE GENE ASSOCIATION STUDIES

Inherent to the success of this approach is the accuracy of selection of the gene of interest. Prior identification of a gene through either linkage studies or thorough knowledge of the pathogenesis enhances the likelihood of success. For MD, several attempts have been made to link genetics with pathophysiology based on analysis of suspect genes, although all have been selected based on a theory of pathogenesis rather than a known physiologic aberration (**Table 3**). The studies are narrowly focused in genetic terms, analyzing from 1 to 39 genes in the candidate pool. Obviously, not all genes will have an equal probability of association with an inner ear disorder, yet it would be extremely fortuitous to correctly identify an important gene without some substantial information indicating a causative role. All of the studies listed find significance for a marker in a candidate gene; however, the importance or accuracy of any of these findings must be placed in context. None of the findings have been replicated in a second population sample, but if this is achieved, it would substantiate the initial claim of association.

Methodology of an association must be scrutinized. Doi and colleagues[58] examined a single SNP in *KCNE1* and *KCNE3* on the hypothesis that these ion transporters are critical to the development of MD. Analysis of these control groups found that they are not in Hardy Weinberg equilibrium, presumably indicating an inadequate control.[59] The reference population is expected to display correct allele sorting, whereas the disease group containing the suspect allele is likely to show substantial disequilibrium, confirming association between genotype and disease of interest. Genotyping errors or population bias must be assumed, and therefore both associations proposed by Doi and colleagues are rejected. The SNP rs1805127 in *KCNE1* tested by Vrabec and colleagues[60] also failed to confirm an association.

Teggi and colleagues[61] claim significance for a mutation-inducing polymorphism in adducin-1(*ADD1*), designated rs4961. Their data indicate significance the minor allele is assumed to cause disease in heterozygotes. Several studies have addressed the association of this SNP in hypertension, in which heterozygous individuals do manifest changes in sodium excretion and blood pressure distinct from individuals without the

Table 3
Single nucleotide polymorphism–based association studies

Gene/SNP	AFD	P	OR	HWDc	Conf	Risk	Assoc Dz
HCFC1							None
rs2266886	29/10	.003	0.26	No	No	Prevents	
rs17421	24/6	.004	0.21	No	No	Prevents	
rs59607260	24/8	.014	0.27	No	No	Prevents	
rs762653	21/9	.015	0.33	No	No	Prevents	
HSPA1A							Parkinson's disease, stroke, NIHL
rs1043618	17/33	.002	3.5	No	No	Causes	
ADD1							Hypertension, stroke, myocardial infarction
rs4961	17/29	.035	2.8	No	No	Causes	
KCNE1							Jervell Lange Nielsen
rs1805127	14/34	—	—	Yes	NC	Causes	
KCNE3	—	—		Yes	No	Causes	

Abbreviations: AFD, allele frequency difference expressed as minor allele frequency (MAF) in controls/MAF in Meniere's disease cases; OR, odds ratio; HWDc, Hardy Weinberg disequilibrium in controls; Conf, confirmed in independent population sample; NC, not confirmed in follow-up study; Assoc Dz, other diseases associated with this single nucleotide polymorphism; NIHL, noise-induced hearing loss; SNP, single nucleotide polymorphism.

mutation. This *ADD1* mutation was previously linked to hypertension, myocardial infarction, and stroke.[62] However, an increased risk for these disorders is not recognized in patients with MD. Because an animal model of adducing-associated hypertension exists, it will be interesting to see future reports of hearing and temporal bone histology from these animals.

Kawaguchi and colleagues[63] examine two SNPs in heat shock 70kD protein 1A (*HSPA1A*), finding significance for one (rs1043618) but not the other (rs1008438). Both SNPs have been widely investigated, and associations with heart disease, stroke, open angle glaucoma, Parkinson's disease, longevity, and noise-induced hearing loss are all reported.[64,65] Once again, a lack of clinical correlation exists between the other diseases associated with these SNPs and MD. Therefore, for both *HSPA1A* and *ADD1* mutations, the altered function that results is not expected to independently cause MD, but rather acts in concert with other unidentified factors to produce the disease.

Vrabec and colleagues[60] examined a series of SNPs in multiple genes broadly selected among several different theories of pathogenesis. The most significant finding was a protective effect of the minor allele in multiple SNPs in the same haplotype block on the X chromosome that includes host cell factor C1 (*HCFC1*). This gene was chosen for its role in herpes virus replication in neurons. Implicit in the association between *HCFC1* and MD is that herpes viruses are potentially a trigger for activation of a molecular pathway that leads to the development of cochleovestibular symptoms.

All of the candidate genes examined could be plausibly linked to MD, and each manuscript outlines a mechanism of disease development that is feasible. The associations are not necessarily exclusive of each other, and therefore the accuracy of these associations relies on replication in subsequent studies.

SUMMARY

Genetic studies of MD have been inconclusive, and therefore fail to enhance understanding of the pathophysiology of the disorder. However, the efforts have been less intensive than for other common diseases such as migraine. The potential for this avenue of investigation to yield important insight is high, and therefore efforts continue. Familial cases account for only a small portion of cases of MD and the genetic basis for the disease may be different in these families. In familial hemiplegic migraine, for example, the genes identified have not yet been found to be significantly associated with common migraine. However, the value of identifying a gene that would lead to a better understanding of the pathogenesis is immense.

As costs for genome-wide scanning decrease, the application of a hypothesis blind approach becomes appealing. Genome-wide scans have the potential to enhance suspicion of a given physiologic mechanism of disease or identify previously unsuspected molecular pathways.

However, important limitations of genome-wide association studies must be considered.[66] The greatest obstacle to genetic investigation using association studies is subject selection. Criteria for diagnosing MD have been established, but these are almost entirely based on clinical history. The only objective evidence available is low-frequency sensorineural hearing loss, although this is hardly specific for MD. Subject accrual will be influenced by the rigidity of inclusion criteria. The more specific the criteria, the longer it will take to amass the necessary sample. However, more rigid entry criteria improve the probability of correctly matching genetic variants with clinical phenotypes.

SNP-based scans using frequently observed polymorphisms are most likely to detect common sequence variants associated with disease development.[57] The effect size of these common variants has been small, usually producing a mildly increased risk for disease development (odds ratio, <2). Experience in other common diseases also shows that a common genetic variant will not account for the entire heritability of the disorder. This observation leads to investigations of rare variants, copy number variation, and epigenetic causes to explain the entire heritability of a given disease.[67,68] Rare structural variants are suspected to account for the molecular differences underlying varied clinical phenotypes.

Ultimately, definition of genetic markers of disease is confirmed through experimental modeling that confirms physiologic dysfunction. Discovery of a mechanism of disease development will advance accuracy of the diagnosis and refinement of clinical phenotypes, and provide new targets for pharmacologic intervention.

REFERENCES

1. Committee on Hearing and Equilibrium guidelines for the diagnosis and evaluation of therapy in Meniere's disease. Otolaryngol Head Neck Surg 1995;113:181–5.
2. Vrabec JT, Simon LM, Coker NJ. Survey of Ménière's disease in a subspecialty referral practice. Otolaryngol Head Neck Surg 2007;137:213–7.
3. House JW, Doherty JK, Fisher LM, et al. Meniere's disease: prevalence of contralateral ear involvement. Otol Neurotol 2006;27:355–61.
4. Silverstein H, Smouha E, Jones R. Natural history vs. surgery for Ménière's disease. Otolaryngol Head Neck Surg 1989;100:6–16.
5. Wladislavosky-Waserman P, Facer GW, Mokri B, et al. Ménière's disease: a 30-year epidemiologic and clinical study in Rochester, MN, 1951–1980. Laryngoscope 1984;94:1098–102.
6. Green JD Jr, Blum DJ, Harner SG. Longitudinal followup of patients with Ménière's disease. Otolaryngol Head Neck Surg 1991;104:783–8.
7. Friberg U, Stahle J, Svedberg A. The natural course of Ménière's disease. Acta Otolaryngol Suppl 1984;406:72–7.
8. Torok N. Old and new in Meniere disease. Laryngoscope 1977;87:1870–7.
9. Ruckenstein MJ, Rutka JA, Hawke M. The treatment of Ménière's disease: Torok revisited. Laryngoscope 1991;101:211–8.
10. Grant IL, Welling DB. The treatment of hearing loss in Ménière's disease. Otolaryngol Clin North Am 1997;30:1123–44.
11. Merchant SN, Adams JC, Nadol JB Jr. Pathophysiology of Meniere's syndrome: are symptoms caused by endolymphatic hydrops? Otol Neurotol 2005;26:74–81.
12. Wangemann P. K+ cycling and the endocochlear potential. Hear Res 2002;165: 1–9.
13. Rauch SD, Zurakowski D, Bloch DB, et al. Anti-heat shock protein 70 antibodies in Ménière's disease. Laryngoscope 2000;110:1516–21.
14. Ruckenstein MJ, Prasthoffer A, Bigelow DC, et al. Immunologic and serologic testing in patients with Ménière's disease. Otol Neurotol 2002;23:517–20.
15. Lempert T, Neuhauser H. Epidemiology of vertigo, migraine and vestibular migraine. J Neurol 2009;256:333–8.
16. Lempert T, Neuhauser H. Migrainous vertigo. Neurol Clin 2005;23:715–30.
17. Battista RA. Audiometric findings of patients with migraine-associated dizziness. Otol Neurotol 2004;25:987–92.
18. Radtke A, Lempert T, Gresty MA, et al. Migraine and Ménière's disease: is there a link? Neurology 2002;59:1700–4.
19. Bikhazi P, Jackson C, Ruckenstein MJ. Efficacy of antimigrainous therapy in the treatment of migraine-associated dizziness. Am J Otol 1997;18:350–4.

20. de Vries B, Frants RR, Ferrari MD, et al. Molecular genetics of migraine. Hum Genet 2009;126:115–32.

21. Vrabec JT. Herpes simplex virus and Ménière's disease. Laryngoscope 2003; 113:1431–8.

22. Ship II, Miller MF, Ram C. A retrospective study of recurrent herpes labialis (RHL) in a professional population, 1958–1971. Oral Surg Oral Med Oral Pathol 1977; 44:723–30.

23. Spruance SL. The natural history of recurrent oral-facial herpes simplex virus infection. Semin Dermatol 1992;11:200–6.

24. Morrison AW, Johnson KJ. Genetics (molecular biology) and Meniere's disease. Otolaryngol Clin North Am 2002;35:497–516.

25. Brown M. Meniere's syndrome. Arch Neurol Psychiatry 1941;46:561–5.

26. Morrison AW. Anticipation in Meniere's disease. J Laryngol Otol 1995;109: 499–502.

27. Bernstein JM. Occurrence of episodic vertigo and hearing loss in families. Ann Otol Rhinol Laryngol 1965;74:1011–21.

28. Birgerson L, Gustavson KH, Stahle J. Familial Ménière's disease: a genetic investigation. Am J Otol 1987;8:323–6.

29. Martini A. Hereditary Ménière's disease: report of two families. Am J Otolaryngol 1982;3:163–7.

30. Fung K, Xie Y, Hall SF, et al. Genetic basis of familial Ménière's disease. J Otolaryngol 2002;31:1–4.

31. Arweiler DJ, Jahnke K, Grosse-Wilde H. Meniere disease as an autosome dominant hereditary disease. Laryngorhinootologie 1995;74:512–5.

32. Oliveira CA, Ferrari I, Messias CI. Occurrence of familial Ménière's syndrome and migraine in Brasilia. Ann Otol Rhinol Laryngol 2002;111: 229–36.

33. Klockars T, Kentala E. Inheritance of Meniere's disease in the Finnish population. Arch Otolaryngol Head Neck Surg 2007;133:73–7.

34. Hilgert N, Smith RJ, Van Camp G. Forty-six genes causing nonsyndromic hearing impairment: which ones should be analyzed in DNA diagnostics? Mutat Res 2009;681:189–96.

35. Xenellis J, Morrison AW, McClowskey D, et al. HLA antigens in the pathogenesis of Ménière's disease. J Laryngol Otol 1986;100:21–4.

36. Koyama S, Mitsuishi Y, Bibee K, et al. HLA associations with Ménière's disease. Acta Otolaryngol 1993;113(5):575–8.

37. López-Escámez JA, López-Nevot A, Cortes R, et al. Expression of A, B, C and DR antigens in definite Meniere's disease in a Spanish population. Eur Arch Otorhinolaryngol 2002;259:347–50.

38. Melchiorri L, Martini A, Rizzo R, et al. Human leukocyte antigen-A, -B, -C and -DR alleles and soluble human leukocyte antigen class I serum level in Ménière's disease. Acta Otolaryngol Suppl 2002;548:26–9.

39. Fransen E, Verstreken M, Verhagen WI, et al. High prevalence of symptoms of Meniere's disease in three families with a mutation in the COCH gene. Hum Mol Genet 1999;8:1425–9.

40. Khetarpal U. DFNA9 is a progressive audiovestibular dysfunction with a microfibrillar deposit in the inner ear. Laryngoscope 2000;110:1379–84.

41. Sanchez E, Lopez-Escamez JA, Lopez-Nevot MA, et al. Absence of COCH mutations in patients with Meniere disease. Eur J Hum Genet 2004;12:75–8.

42. Frykholm C, Larsen HC, Dahl N, et al. Familial Meniere's disease in five generations. Otol Neurotol 2006;27:681–6.

43. Klar J, Frykholm C, Friberg U, et al. A Meniere's disease gene linked to chromosome 12p12.3. Am J Med Genet B Neuropsychiatr Genet 2006;141:463–7.
44. Lynch M, Cameron TL, Knight M, et al. Structural and mutational analysis of antiquitin as a candidate gene for Meniere disease. Am J Med Genet 2002;110: 397–9.
45. Mhatre AN, Jero J, Chiappini I, et al. Aquaporin-2 expression in the mammalian cochlea and investigation of its role in Meniere's disease. Hear Res 2002;170: 59–69.
46. Kimura RS. Animal models of endolymphatic hydrops. Am J Otolaryngol 1982;3: 447–51.
47. Horner KC. Auditory and vestibular function in experimental hydrops. Otolaryngol Head Neck Surg 1995;112:84–9.
48. Xia AP, Kikuchi T, Minowa O, et al. Late-onset hearing loss in a mouse model of DFN3 non-syndromic deafness: morphologic and immunohistochemical analyses. Hear Res 2002;166:150–8.
49. Yang T, Vidarsson H, Rodrigo-Blomqvist S, et al. Transcriptional control of SLC26A4 is involved in Pendred syndrome and nonsyndromic enlargement of vestibular aqueduct (DFNB4). Am J Hum Genet 2007;80:1055–63.
50. Megerian CA, Semaan MT, Aftab S, et al. A mouse model with postnatal endolymphatic hydrops and hearing loss. Hear Res 2008;237:90–105.
51. Meister M, Johnson A, Popelka GR, et al. Audiologic findings in young patients with hypophosphatemic bone disease. Ann Otol Rhinol Laryngol 1986;95:415–20.
52. Risch N, Merikangas K. The future of genetic studies of complex human diseases. Science 1996;273(5281):1516–7.
53. Botstein D, Risch N. Discovering genotypes underlying human phenotypes: past successes for Mendelian disease, future approaches for complex disease. Nat Genet 2003;33(Suppl):228–37.
54. Ke X, Hunt S, Tapper W, et al. The impact of SNP density on fine-scale patterns of linkage disequilibrium. Hum Mol Genet 2004;13:577–88.
55. Cardon LR, Bell JI. Association study designs for complex diseases. Nat Rev Genet 2001;2:91–9.
56. Becker N, Nieters A, Rittgen W. Single nucleotide polymorphism–disease relationships: statistical issues for the performance of association studies. Mutat Res 2003;525:11–8.
57. Zondervan KT, Cardon LR. The complex interplay among factors that influence allelic association. Nat Rev Genet 2004;5:89–100.
58. Doi K, Sato T, Kuramasu T, et al. Ménière's disease is associated with single nucleotide polymorphisms in the human potassium channel genes, KCNE1 and KCNE3. ORL J Otorhinolaryngol Relat Spec 2005;67:289–93.
59. Hoh J, Wille A, Ott J. Trimming, weighting, and grouping SNPs in human case-control association studies. Genome Res 2001;11:2115–9.
60. Vrabec JT, Liu L, Li B, et al. Sequence variants in host cell factor C1 are associated with Ménière's disease. Otol Neurotol 2008;29:561–6.
61. Teggi R, Lanzani C, Zagato L, et al. Gly460Trp alpha-adducin mutation as a possible mechanism leading to endolymphatic hydrops in Ménière's syndrome. Otol Neurotol 2008;29:824–8.
62. Bianchi G, Ferrari P, Staessen JA. Adducin polymorphism detection and impact on hypertension. Hypertension 2005;45:331–40.
63. Kawaguchi S, Hagiwara A, Suzuki M. Polymorphic analysis of the heat-shock protein 70 gene (HSPA1A) in Ménière's disease. Acta Otolaryngol 2008;128: 1173–7.

64. Wu YR, Wang CK, Chen CM, et al. Analysis of heat-shock protein 70 gene poly-morphisms and the risk of Parkinson's disease. Hum Genet 2004;114:236–41.

65. Konings A, Van Laer L, Michel S, et al. Variations in HSP70 genes associated with noise-induced hearing loss in two independent populations. Eur J Hum Genet 2009;17:329–35.

66. Frazer KA, Murray SS, Schork NJ, et al. Human genetic variation and its contribu-tion to complex traits. Nat Rev Genet 2009;10:241–51.

67. Schork NJ, Murray SS, Frazer KA, et al. Common vs. rare allele hypotheses for complex diseases. Curr Opin Genet Dev 2009;19:212–9.

68. Wong KK, deLeeuw RJ, Dosanjh NS, et al. A comprehensive analysis of common copy-number variations in the human genome. Am J Hum Genet 2007;80: 91–104.

Erratum:
Dr. Aldo Stamm,
Lead Author

In the June 2010 issue of Otolaryngologic Clinics, *Rhinology: Evolution of Science and Surgery*, please note misappropriation of authors in the article, "Evolution of Endoscopic Skull Base Surgery, Current Concepts, and Future Perspectives." The senior lead and corresponding author is **Dr. Aldo Stamm**. Director of the São Paulo ENT Center and Hospital Prof. Edmundo Vasconcelos, São Paulo, Brazil. astamm@terra.com.br.

Otolaryngol Clin N Am 43 (2010) 1133
doi:10.1016/j.otc.2010.07.001
0030-6665/10/$ – see front matter © 2010 Elsevier Inc. All rights reserved.

INDEX

Note: Page numbers of article titles are in **boldface** type.

Otolaryngol Clin N Am 43 (2010) 1135–1141
doi:10.1016/S0030-6665(10)00168-4
0030-6665/10/$ – see front matter © 2010 Elsevier Inc. All rights reserved.

oto.theclinics.com

United States Postal Service

Statement of Ownership, Management, and Circulation
(All Periodicals Publications Except Requestor Publications)

1. Publication Title
Otolaryngologic Clinics of North America

2. Publication Number
4 6 6 - 5 5 0

3. Filing Date
9/15/10

4. Issue Frequency
Feb, Apr, Jun, Aug, Oct, Dec

5. Number of Issues Published Annually
6

6. Annual Subscription Price
$290.00

7. Complete Mailing Address of Known Office of Publication *(Not printer) (Street, city, county, state, and ZIP+4®)*

Elsevier Inc.
360 Park Avenue South
New York, NY 10010-1710

Contact Person
Stephen Bushing

Telephone *(Include area code)*
215-239-3688

8. Complete Mailing Address of Headquarters or General Business Office of Publisher *(Not printer)*

Elsevier Inc., 360 Park Avenue South, New York, NY 10010-1710

9. Full Names and Complete Mailing Addresses of Publisher, Editor, and Managing Editor *(Do not leave blank)*

Publisher *(Name and complete mailing address)*

Kim Murphy, Elsevier, Inc., 1600 John F. Kennedy Blvd. Suite 1800, Philadelphia, PA 19103-2899

Editor *(Name and complete mailing address)*

Joanne Husovski, Elsevier, Inc., 1600 John F. Kennedy Blvd. Suite 1800, Philadelphia, PA 19103-2899

Managing Editor *(Name and complete mailing address)*

Catherine Bewick, Elsevier, Inc., 1600 John F. Kennedy Blvd. Suite 1800, Philadelphia, PA 19103-2899

10. Owner *(Do not leave blank. If the publication is owned by a corporation, give the name and address of the corporation immediately followed by the names and addresses of all stockholders owning or holding 1 percent or more of the total amount of stock. If not owned by a corporation, give the names and addresses of the individual owners. If owned by a partnership or other unincorporated firm, give its name and address as well as those of each individual owner. If the publication is published by a nonprofit organization, give its name and address.)*

Full Name	Complete Mailing Address
Wholly owned subsidiary of	4520 East-West Highway
Reed/Elsevier, US holdings	Bethesda, MD 20814

11. Known Bondholders, Mortgagees, and Other Security Holders Owning or Holding 1 Percent or More of Total Amount of Bonds, Mortgages, or Other Securities. If none, check box. ☐ None

Full Name	Complete Mailing Address
N/A	

12. Tax Status *(For completion by nonprofit organizations authorized to mail at nonprofit rates) (Check one)*
The purpose, function, and nonprofit status of this organization and the exempt status for Federal income tax purposes:
☐ Has Not Changed During Preceding 12 Months
☐ Has Changed During Preceding 12 Months *(Publisher must submit explanation of change with this statement)*

PS Form 3526, September 2007 (Page 1 of 3 (Instructions Page 3)) PSN 7530-01-000-9931 PRIVACY NOTICE: See our Privacy policy in www.usps.com

---

13. Publication Title
Otolaryngologic Clinics of North America

14. Issue Date for Circulation Data Below
August 2010

15. Extent and Nature of Circulation

		Average No. Copies Each Issue During Preceding 12 Months	No. Copies of Single Issue Published Nearest to Filing Date
a. Total Number of Copies *(Net press run)*		2385	2200
b. Paid Circulation (By Mail and Outside the Mail)	(1) Mailed Outside-County Paid Subscriptions Stated on PS Form 3541. *(Include paid distribution above nominal rate, advertiser's proof copies, and exchange copies)*	927	860
	(2) Mailed In-County Paid Subscriptions Stated on PS Form 3541 *(Include paid distribution above nominal rate, advertiser's proof copies, and exchange copies)*		
	(3) Paid Distribution Outside the Mails Including Sales Through Dealers and Carriers, Street Vendors, Counter Sales, and Other Paid Distribution Outside USPS®	732	622
	(4) Paid Distribution by Other Classes Mailed Through the USPS (e.g. First-Class Mail®)		
c. Total Paid Distribution *(Sum of 15b (1), (2), (3), and (4))*	▲	1659	1482
d. Free or Nominal Rate Distribution (By Mail and Outside the Mail)	(1) Free or Nominal Rate Outside-County Copies Included on PS Form 3541	100	107
	(2) Free or Nominal Rate In-County Copies Included on PS Form 3541		
	(3) Free or Nominal Rate Copies Mailed at Other Classes Through the USPS (e.g. First-Class Mail)		
	(4) Free or Nominal Rate Distribution Outside the Mail (Carriers or other means)		
e. Total Free or Nominal Rate Distribution *(Sum of 15d (1), (2), (3) and (4))*	▲	100	107
f. Total Distribution *(Sum of 15c and 15e)*	▲	1759	1589
g. Copies not Distributed *(See instructions to publishers #4 (page #3))*	▲	626	611
h. Total *(Sum of 15f and g)*	▲	2385	2200
i. Percent Paid *(15c divided by 15f times 100)*		94.31%	93.27%

16. Publication of Statement of Ownership
☐ If the publication is a general publication, publication of this statement is required. Will be printed in the October 2010 issue of this publication. ☐ Publication not required

17. Signature and Title of Editor, Publisher, Business Manager, or Owner

Stephen R. Bushing — Fulfillment/Inventory Specialist

Date September 15, 2010

I certify that all information furnished on this form is true and complete. I understand that anyone who furnishes false or misleading information on this form or who omits material or information requested on the form may be subject to criminal sanctions (including fines and imprisonment) and/or civil sanctions (including civil penalties).

PS Form 3526, September 2007 (Page 2 of 3)

Moving?

Make sure your subscription moves with you!

To notify us of your new address, find your **Clinics Account Number** (located on your mailing label above your name), and contact customer service at:

Email: journalscustomerservice-usa@elsevier.com

800-654-2452 (subscribers in the U.S. & Canada)
314-447-8871 (subscribers outside of the U.S. & Canada)

Fax number: 314-447-8029

Elsevier Health Sciences Division
Subscription Customer Service
3251 Riverport Lane
Maryland Heights, MO 63043

*To ensure uninterrupted delivery of your subscription,
please notify us at least 4 weeks in advance of move.

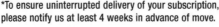

Printed and bound by CPI Group (UK) Ltd, Croydon, CR0 4YY

03/10/2024

01040453-0017